Cancer in the First Year of Life

Contributions to Oncology
Beiträge zur Onkologie

Vol. 41

Series Editors
J. H. Holzner, Wien; *W. Queißer,* Mannheim

KARGER

Basel · München · Paris · London · New York · New Delhi · Bangkok · Singapore · Tokyo · Sydney

Cancer in the First Year of Life

Leukemias; Neuroblastomas; Soft Tissue Sarcomas

Volume Editors

F. Lampert, Gießen, *L. Cordero di Montezemolo,* Turin; *A. Pession,* Bologna

53 figures und 65 tables, 1990

KARGER

Basel · München · Paris · London · New York · New Delhi · Bangkok · Singapore · Tokyo · Sydney

Contributions to Oncology
Beiträge zur Onkologie

Drug Dosage
The authors and the publisher have exerted every effort to ensure that drug selection and dosage set forth in this text are in accord with current recommendations and practice at the time of publication. However, in view of ongoing research, changes in government regulations, and the constant flow of information relating to drug therapy and drug reactions, the reader is urged to check the package insert for each drug for any change in indications and dosage and for added warnings and precautions. This is particularly important when the recommended agent is a new and/or infrequently employed drug.

© Copyright 1990 by S. Karger GmbH, P.O. Box 1724, D-8034 Germering/München and
S. Karger AG, Postfach, CH-4009 Basel
Printed in Germany by Bonitas-Bauer, Würzburg
ISBN 3-8055-5233-5

Contents

Contents

Preface

The purpose of this volume is twofold: 1) Selecting a topic which deserves more attention, namely Cancer in the First Year of Life, concentrating mainly on leukemias, neuroblastomas and soft tissue sarcomas, and 2) documenting an example of Italo-German collaboration in the field of pediatric cancer.

In 1985 at a meeting in Cologne, the Bilateral Agreement Italy – Federal Republic of Germany, funded by the Consiglio Nazionale delle Ricerche, Progetto Finalizzato 'Oncologia' and the Deutsche Forschungsgemeinschaft, was started, and pediatric oncology was one of the fields included. In the meantime, there were many bilateral activities, including exchange of diagnostic and therapy protocols and also laboratory and clinical personnel. So far, several Italian scientists from Italy have stayed at laboratories (Giessen, Göttingen, Heidelberg) for up to 6 months. Genoa was the host of the first Workshop of Pathologists in December 1987, and the first Workshop on Pediatric Oncology in November 1987, focusing on metastatic neuroblastoma, rhabdomyosarcoma, histiocytoses, B-cell disease. The idea of joined efforts was to have either combined studies in rare tumor diseases or parallel studies in common malignancies in order to gain more knowledge and to cure more children.

Thus, a second Italo-German Workshop on Pediatric Oncology (with 34 Italian and 25 German participants) took place October 27/28, 1989, at Braunfels, an ancient Hessian town in the Taunus mountains, and had only one sole topic: Cancer in the newborn and infant. 35 papers were presented, regarding epidemiology, diagnosis, therapy, general management of malignancies in infancy, particulary leukemias, neuroblastoma, soft tissue tumors. Due to space limitations in this volume we had to omit contributions on general aspects; and in some instances only abstracts with some tables or diagrams could be printed. It was anticipated, however, that Italian and German papers should alternate, often on the same subject.

Some results of the workshop can be summarized: Cancer incidence was found to be higher in infants as compared to age groups of older children, and neuroblastoma was the most frequent tumor. Leukemias, on the other hand, occur more rarely and, in ALL, have a poorer therapy response in infants as compared to older children. The immunophenotypes of leukemic cells in infancy are different as are the genotypes, with translocation t(4;11) being the most common one. Clinical and cytological peculiarities are seen in the Transient Myeloproliferative Disorders, often affecting newborns with Down's syndrome, and in these cases intensive therapy should be restricted. Neuroblastomas in infants could be evaluated as to prognostic factors, and the high number of low stage patients was found to be responsible for the high survival rate in infancy. It was possible to demonstrate that 1p-aberrations and copy number of the oncogene N-myc were the most important cytogenetic predictors. Cytogenetic investigations in families with a neuroblastoma patient pointed to a certain disposition for tumor occurrence. Highlight of the workshop was the guest lecture of Thomas Boehm from the MRC Laboratory of Molecular Biology, Cambridge, who demonstrated how breakpoints on the short arm of chromosome 11 in cells of T-acute lymphoblastic leukemia could be located, sequenced, and explained in their gene expression.

Gießen / Genoa, August 1990   *Fritz Lampert*
                                                                     Luisa Massimo

Contrib Oncol. Basel, Karger, 1990, vol 41, pp 1–7.

Epidemiological Data on Childhood Malignancies in the First Year of Life

P. Kaatsch, J. Michaelis

Institute for Medical Statistics and Documentation, University of Mainz, FRG

Zusammenfassung

Im Mainzer Kinderkrebsregister wurden von 1980 bis 1988 bundesweit 1.336 bösartige Erkrankungen bei Kindern im ersten Lebensjahr erfaßt. In der vorliegenden Arbeit werden einige Charakteristika dieser Patienten denen der übrigen Patienten im Kindesalter gegenübergestellt. Mit 20,9 Neuerkrankungen pro 100.000 Kinder ist die Inzidenz im ersten Lebensjahr im Vergleich zu den übrigen Altersklassen des Kindesalters am höchsten. Das Krankheitsspektrum weicht deutlich von dem der älteren Kinder ab, am häufigsten sind die Tumoren des sympathischen Nervensystems, gefolgt von ZNS-Tumoren und Leukämien. Auch die Überlebenskurven der im ersten Lebensjahr erkrankten Kinder unterscheiden sich deutlich von denen des übrigen Kindesalters, was ein Hinweis auf Unterschiede in der Tumorbiologie sein kann.

Introduction

Since 1980, a nationwide registry of childhood malignancies in the FRG is run at the 'Institut für Medizinische Statistik und Dokumentation' (IMSD) in Mainz. Based on a concerted action of the two German scientific societies of pediatric oncology, GPO and DAL, more than 100 pediatric hospitals and centers of pediatric oncology are reporting all their cancer patients to the registry on a voluntary basis. It is estimated that with an annual registration of approximately 1,200 newly diseased children, more than 95 % of the total incidence is covered by the registry [1]. Thereby, according to a recent publication from the International Agency for Research on Cancer [2], the registry is at present the largest single registry of childhood malignancies. The mentioned publication contains data from more than 60 registries, and a comparison shows that, with the exception of the CNS tumors, our estimated incidences are in a similar range as in other large registries.

On the occasion of the Italian-German symposium on cancer in the first year of life, a special evaluation of our registry was performed, based on all cases reported from 1980 to 1988.

Material and Methods

Following admission of a newly diseased individual to one of the cooperating hospitals, a notification form is sent to our registry. This form contains patient identification data, a tentative diagnosis and the information whether the patient will be included in one of the 15 ongoing clinical trials organized by the GPO and DAL. In response to the notification, the IMSD sends a set of tumor-specific documentation forms to the cooperating clinician. If the patient takes part in a clinical trial, which is the case in about 65 % of all patients, the documentation on the tumor-specific forms is checked by the trial centers, which also collect the follow-up informations for at least 5 years after the beginning of the treatment. Data exchange between the trial centers and the registry is based on microcomputers with software centrally developed at our institute [3]. The collection of follow-up information on non-trial patients and on all patients beyond the time span of the clinical trials is organized by the IMSD.

Integration of data from clinical trials into the central registry enhances both the quality and completeness of data and increases the speed of availability. Additionally, it allows the storage of more information than is usually kept in cancer registries, which can be used for additional studies like analysis of late effects of therapy. The present evaluation is based on the data on 10,167 children below 15 years of age which were registered between 1980 and 1988. For the disease-specific analyses we used the classification proposed by Birch and Marsden [4].

Results

Incidence and Disease Spectrum

Calculation of incidence rates is based on the cases registered in the years 1983 to 1987 because the data were incomplete in the first years of operation of the registry, and population data have not yet been made available for 1988 for the FRG. Whereas the incidence of all childhood malignancies is estimated as 12.6 per 100,000 children with age below 15 years, the incidence during the first year of life is 20.9, which is the highest incidence in total childhood. Figure 1 shows the incidence in infants to be nearly as high as in the age group for 1 to 4 years and about half as high in later age groups. The proportion of boys among all diseased children is 56.7 % and during the first year of life only 53.3 %. The incidence per 100,000 for boys in the first year is 22.3, and for girls 19.5.

The age-specific incidences for the different diseases show marked differences. Figure 2 give some representative examples: The one extreme is the neuroblastoma with the highest incidence of all tumors in infants (5.1/100,000). The acute lymphoblastic leukemia shows a peak at the third and fourth year of life. In contrast, there are some diseases, like Hodgkin's disease or bone tumors, which hardly ever occur in infants. A comparison of the relative frequency of malignancies occuring in the first year of life with the disease spectrum which is observed in the later years of childhood is shown in figure 3. Among 1,336 children below one year of age, tumors of the sympathetic nervous system were most frequent (21,9 %) followed by tumors of the CNS and leukemias with a percentage of 15–16 %. Among 8,831 children with age from one to 14 years, leukemias are most frequent (38,4 %), followed by CNS tumors and lymphomas with other reticuloendothelial neoplasms, with about 15 % each. Germ cell, trophoblastic and other gonadal neoplasms are more than five times as frequent in the first year of life than in years 3 to 14.

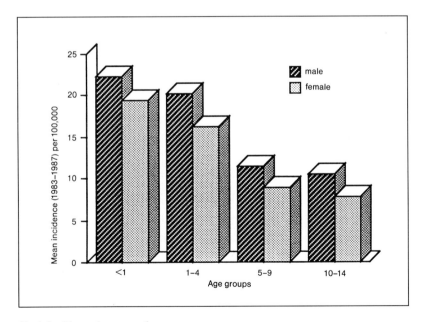

Fig 1. Incidence by sex and age groups.

Survival analysis

Follow-up information was available for 784 patients whose disease started in the first year of life, and 7,542 patients who developed their disease from one to 14 years of age. In figure 4, the Kaplan-Meier curves for these overall groups are presented. One can see that the survival rates are lower for the younger children up to a follow-up of about 4 years when both curves reach a kind of plateau close to 75 %. The analysis of the acute lymphoblastic leukemia is shown in figure 5, and one can see that survival is much worse for the children diseased in the first year of life, with a five-

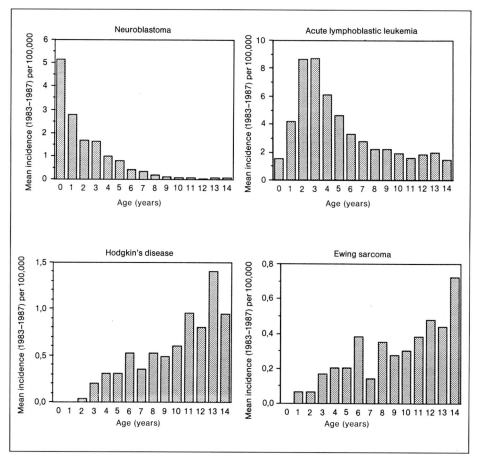

Fig 2. Age-specific incidences for selected diagnoses.

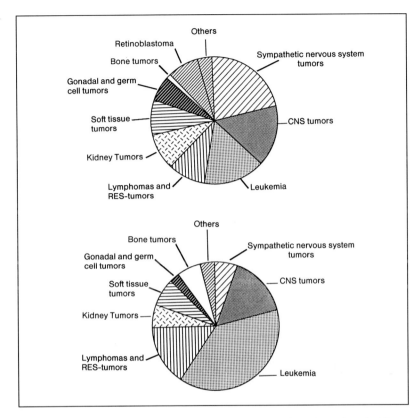

Fig 3. Disease spectrum for the children below one year of age (above) and with age from one to 14 years (below).

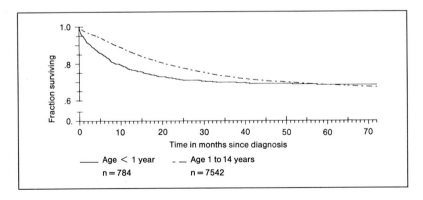

Fig 4. Overall survival curve (Kaplan-Meier).

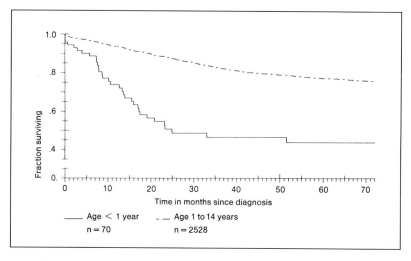

Fig 5. Survival curve for acute lymphoblastic leukemia (Kaplan-Meier).

year-survival rate of 44 %, compared to the survival of the elder children, with 77 % after five years. Also, the prognosis of CNS tumors is worse for the younger children. The contrary is the case for tumors of the sympathetic nervous system. This corresponds to the well-known fact of good prognosis of neuroblastoma in the first year of life.

Discussion and Outlook

The paper gives an overview of the occurence of cancer in the first year of life, based on 1,336 cases which were collected from 1980–1988 in the nationwide registry of childhood malignancies of the FRG. It thereby provides some basic information about malignant diseases in infants, to which selected aspects were presented in more detail on the occasion of the Italian-German symposium by the principial investigators of special clinical trials and other experts.

Since the registry includes a continuous follow-up of all patients, we were also able to perform survival analyses. With respect to the prognosis, the presented survival curves give a global impression of the course of different diseases which started in the first year of life as compared to a beginning in the later childhood. Further analysis, e. g. with respect to histological diagnosis and tumor stages, has to be performed. However, already the epidemiological overview suggests that tumors developing in the first year of life are associated with other biological behaviour than tumors occurring later in childhood.

Summary

From 1980 to 1988, 1336 children diseased in the first year of life were reported to the registry of childhood malignancies in the FRG. This corresponds to an annual incidence of 20.9/100,000 and is the highest incidence in childhood. The disease pattern in the first year of life is different from later childhood. Most frequent are tumours of the sympathetic nervous system (21.9 %), followed by tumours of the CNS (16 %) and leukemias (15 %). For some tumour entities, survival rates also differ between diseases in the first year of life and later childhood and thus may indicate differences in tumour biology.

References

1   Michaelis J, Kaatsch P: Cooperative documentation of childhood malignancies in the FRG – System design and five-year results in Riehm H (ed): Monogr Paediat. Basel, Karger, 1986, vol 18, pp 56 – 67.
2   Parkin DM, Stiller CA, Draper GJ, Bieber CA, Terracini B, Young JL (eds): International incidence of childhood cancer. Lyon, IARC Scientific publications 87, 1988.
3   Michaelis J, Kaatsch P: Use of information from clinical trials for an integrated cancer registry. Methods Inf Med 1990;29:92 – 98.
4   Birch JM, Marsden HB: A classification scheme for childhood cancer. Int J Cancer 1987;40:620 – 624.

Dipl. Inform. Med. Peter Kaatsch, Institut für Medizinische Statistik und Dokumentation, Klinikum der Johannes-Gutenberg-Universität, Postfach 3960, Langenbeckstr. 1, D-6500 Mainz (FRG)

Contrib Oncol. Basel, Karger, 1990, vol 41, pp 8–9.

Cancer in the First Year of Life: Childhood Cancer Registry of Piedmont, 1967–1986 (Abstract)

R. Colombo[a], *L. Giordano*[b], *M.L. Mosso*[a], *B. Terracini*[b], *G. Pastore*[a], *C. Magnani*[b]

[a] Childhood Cancer Registry of Piedmont
[b] Servizio Universitario di Epidemiologia dei Tumori, Turin, Italy

The Childhood Cancer Registry of Piedmont collects cases of cancer occuring among children aged 0–14, who are residents in Piedmont (Italy).

Incidence and mortality data are available for the period 1967–1986: The total number of cases registered over 20 years in the Province of Torino (the largest province of Piedmont, about 500,000 children in the age 0–14) was 1321, of which 113 were diagnosed in the first year of life.

Table 1. Incidence rates (×1,000,000). Age 0 to 14 years (Province of Torino 1967–1986)

	Males	Females	Total
Leukemias	49.8	41.5	45.8
Tumors of the CNS	33.6	28.6	31.2
Neuroblastomas	11.8	7.9	9.9
Hodgkin's lymphomas	8.1	5.2	6.7
Non-HD lymphomas	12.2	3.7	8.1
Soft tissue sarcomas	9.5	6.6	8.1
Sarcomas of the bone	7.7	8.3	8.0
Renal cancers	6.2	8.1	7.1
Retinoblastomas	3.1	3.1	3.1
Other	12.4	12.8	12.7
Total	154.6	125.8	140.6

Table 2. Incidence rates (×1,000,000) in the first year of life (Province of Torino 1967–1986)

	Males	Females	Total cases	Rates
Leukemias	49.0	45.1	26	47.1
ALL	17.5	15.0	9	16.3
AnLL	14.0	0.0	4	7.3
Other leukemias	17.5	30.1	13	23.6
Tumors of the CNS	17.5	30.1	13	23.6
Medulloblastomas	3.5	7.5	3	5.4
Astrocytomas, ependimomas,				
Glyomas	7.0	3.8	3	5.4
Other	7.0	18.8	7	12.8
Neuroblastomas	45.5	26.3	20	36.3
Lymphomas	7.0	3.8	3	5.4
Soft tissue sarcomas	21.0	15.0	10	18.1
Sarcomas of the bone	0.0	7.5	2	3.6
Renal cancers	10.5	37.6	13	23.6
Retinoblastomas	7.0	22.5	8	14.5
Other	28.0	37.6	18	32.7
Total	185.6	225.5	113	204.9

L. Giordano, Servizio Universitario di Epidemiologia dei Tumori,
Via Santena 7, I-10126 Torino (Italy)

Contrib Oncol. Basel, Karger, 1990, vol 41, pp 10–17.

Acute Lymphoblastic and Non-Lymphoblastic Leukemia in Infants Less Than 1 Year of Age

A Cumulative Experience of the Associazione Italiana Ematologia Oncologia Pediatrica (AIEOP)[1]

C. Guazzelli[a], *A. Rosi*[a], *A. Pession*[b], *R. Rondelli*[b], *A. Lippi*[a],
M. Giuliano[b], *G. Paolucci*[b]

[a] DPTO. Pediatria-Ematologia, Florence
[b] Clinica Pediatrica III – Bologna, Italy

Zusammenfassung

Die Daten von 152 Säuglingen, die von 1975–1989 innerhalb multizentrischerStudien der Italienischen Pädiatrischen Hämato-Onkologischen Gesellschaft behandelt wurden, wurden ausgewertet. 116 (76 %) hatten eine akute lymphoblastische Leukämie (ALL), 36 (24 %) eine akute nicht-lymphoblastische Leukämie (ANLL). Die mittlere initiale Leukozytenzahl betrug 64×10^3 pro μl für die ALL und 36×10^3 pro μl für die ANLL. Der Leukämiekaryotyp konnte bei 24 Patienten bestimmt werden, wobei 10 abnormale auffielen und darunter 4 mit Chromosomen-Translokation t(4;11). Bei den 36 Patienten mit ANLL herrschte die myelomonozytäre (FAB-M$_4$) und monoblastische (FAB-M$_5$) Zellmorphologie vor. Die Überlebenswahrscheinlichkeit nach 5 Jahren betrug 30 % und war nicht abhängig von spezifischen Therapieprotokollen. Die Beginnleukozytenzahl war jedoch prognostisch bedeutsam.

Introduction

Acute lymphoblastic (ALL) and non-Lymphoblastic (ANLL) leukemia are clinically and biologically heterogeneous diseases for which specific therapeutic regimen have been designed.

[1]Participating AIEOP Centers: C. Uderzo (Monza), A. Garaventa (Genoa), A. Loiacono (Bari), L. Nespoli (Pavia), R. Miniero (Torino), L. Zanesco (Padua), A. Russo (Catania), P. Rosito (Bologna), T. Barbui (Bergamo), M. Lo Curto (Palermo), P. A. Macchia (Pisa), G. Digilio (Rome), P.L. Giorgi (Ancona), M.T.Di Tullio (Naples), A. Cimaglia (Naples), A. Amici (Perugia), S. Amadori (Rome), A. Acquaviva (Siena), A. Ugazio (Brescia), R. Corda (Cagliari), G. Torlontano (Pescara), D. Rosati (Rome), Italy

In ALL, numerous factors were found to have a prognostic significance, among which age and initial leukocyte count are the major indicators of outcome and were used to stratify patients for treatment selection.

In contrast to the high cure rate in childhood ALL, a much lower rate is reported in infants less than 1 year of age (60 % versus 20 %). Recent prospective trials of the Childrens' Cancer Study Group (CCSG) and Pediatric Oncology Group (POG) have also demonstrated that fewer than 35 % of infants survived 3 years from diagnosis [1, 2].

In AnLL, as a consequence of the overall poor outcome, the prognostic significance of biologic parameters remain equivocal. Nevertheless, the younger seem to fare worse than the older children; 20 % versus 50 % three-years disease-free survival.

At the time of diagnosis, infants were present with a constellation of clinical features associated with a poor prognosis such as an elevated WBC count, organomegaly and CNS leukemia at diagnosis. In addition, the blasts of infants with ALL more frequently have a common ALL antigen (CALLA) negative phenotype, which also has important prognostic implications.

More recently, increased frequencies have been reported for cytogenetic abnormalities: Pseudodiploidy, hypodiploidy and translocations, a break at the region 11q23. Probably these abnormalities are also responsible for the poorest prognosis of this group of patients, but this relationship must be investigated better [3].

The young age adverse effect may be partially explained by the segregation of known high-risk factors such high and extensive leukemic blast burden at presentation, FAB morphology, immunology, etc. Some investigators attributed the poor outcome to excessive toxicity and suboptimal therapy, whereas others disagree with these observations. In fact, intensive regimens recently introduced may lead to improved results [4].

This retrospective study represent an essential background to define a strategical approach to the treatment of acute leukemia in infants in our country.

Clinical and biological features at diagnosis

This study was undertaken to examine in detail the presentation, response to therapy and clinical outcome of all 152 infants < 12 months of age (5 days to 11 months), 69 female (45.4 %) and 83 male (54.6 %), treated in AIEOP Centers during the 14-year period, 1975 to 1989, with different protocols.

At diagnosis, 116 infants (76 %) were affected by ALL, 36 (24 %) by AnLL. In the ALL group, 59 (51.7 %) were under 6 months of age, 4 out of this subgroup were congenital <29 days at diagnosis. The remaining 57 (49 %) were between 6 and 12 months of age. In the AnLL group 33 % were <6 months of age.

WBC count at time of diagnosis for all 152 patients ranged from 2.5×10^3/mmc to $>1 \times 10^6$/mmc. The median values for WBC count were 64.0×10^3/mmc and 35.5×10^3/mmc for ALL and AnLL respectively. In the ALL group, WBC count was $>100 \times 10^3$/mmc in 38 patients (32.8 %); it ranged from 50 to 99×10^3/mmc in 24 patients (20.7 %), from 10 to 49×10^3/mmc in 31 patients (26.7 %), and in 23 patients (19.8 %) WBC count was $<10 \times 10^3$/mmc (table 1).

CNS leukemia at the time of diagnosis was documented in 4 out of 116 patients with a frequency of 3.5 %. No significant correlation between CNS leukemia at diagnosis and present WBC count existed.

Mediastinal mass (M/T>0.33) was present in 5 out of 116 patients (4.3 %). Massive hepatosplenomegaly (palpable at or below the level of umbilicus) was present in 26.5 % (31/116). The leukemia-lymphoma syndrome (LLS), defined according to CCSG criteria with least one laboratory parameter such as WBC count>50×10^3/mmc, or Hb>10g/dl, T cell phenotype and at least one of the clinical features such as mediastinal mass, bulky adenophaty, massive splenomegaly, was present in 19 out of 116 (16.4 %) at diagnosis.

The French-American-British (FAB) morphology of this group was: L1, 71 patients (61.2 %); L2, 21 patients (18.1 %) and not known, 21 patients (18.1 %). According to the BFM risk index this population is distributed in 67 %<0.8, 13.2 % between 0.8 and 1.2, 19.8>1.2.

A cytogenetic study was performed in 24/116 patients; within this group were 10 patients with abnormalities: 4 t(4,11); 1 t(4,17); 1 t(13,14); 2(21+) Down's syndrome and 2 others. Differences in distribution of characteristics assessed by chi-square tests of homogenity of proportion showed in infants a significancy (p <0.0001) increased incidence of hyperleucocytosis (WBC count $>100 \times 10^3$/mmc), hepatosplenomegaly, and failure to achieve complete remission (CR) (table 2).

In the group of infants with AnLL, 36 patients were studied. Two infants died before any treatment, the remaining 34 patients (15 female, 19 male) entered on the therapeutic protocols (51.2 % on the AIEOP and 48.8 % on the not-AIEOP protocols). At the time of diagnosis, 13 patients (38 %) presented WBC count<20×10^3/mmc, 13 (38 %) with 20 to 99 $\times 10^3$/mmc, and 8 (24 %) with WBC count>100×10^3/mmc. An excess of FAB classification M4 and M5 (myelomonocytic and monoblastic) subtypes, which are associated with a less favorable prognosis, has been observed in infants with AnLL.

Table 1. Clinical features in infants < 1 year of age with ALL

WBC count $\times 10^3$/mmc median (min–max)	60	(2.5–999)
Hb g/dl	7.5	(2.7–16)
Plt. $\times 10^3$/mmc	40	(1–485)
Hepatosplenomegaly ($\geq$ OT)	28	(26.5 %)
Mediastinal mass (M/T $\geq$ 0.33)	5	(4.3 %)
CNS Leukemia	4	(3.5 %)

CNS leukemia at diagnosis was documented in five out of 34 patients with a frequency of 14 %. Among the infants with AnLL entered on our retrospective study, no mediastinal mass or massive hepatosplenomegaly were found. Hyperleucocytosis and skin infiltration were observed in 5 of 34 patients infants (1 FAB M1 and 4 FAB M4/M5) younger than 6 months.

Within this group were 4 patients with Down's syndrome.

Response to Therapy and Complication

Although ALL infants were treated on different protocols, induction chemotherapy was nearly identical in all the series of the AIEOP protocols and consisted of daily prednisone (40 mg/sqm), plus daunomicine (20 mg/sqm) and L-Asparaginase I.M. (6.000 U/Sqm). Differences existed in the group treated with not-AIEOP protocols (n=35) regarding induction chemotherapy, and CNS prophylaxis schedule.

Out of 111 patients evaluable for CR, 88 (79.3 %) successfully completed the induction phase of therapy (table 3).

Major induction failures included an induction death rate of 17 % (19/111) (5 sepsis, 3 cardiac failure, 3 cerebral hemorrhage, 8 others, such as bone marrow aplasia, pneumonia, hepatic failure and progressive disease).

Early disease recurrence, characterized by bone marrow (BM) (n=23) and CNS (n=15) relapse, was the major factor responsible for the poor prognosis of this group. CNS relapses were also observed in those patients who received cranial irradiation as part of CNS prophilaxis.

In the AnLL group, 23 patients (69.7 %) successfully completed the induction phase of therapy. Table 3 demonstrates the progress of all 33 evaluable patients. Major induction toxicities included death rate of 24.2 % (3 induction failures, 2 cardiac failure, 1 sepsis, 1 acute enteritis and 1 not known).

Table 2. Biological characteristics more frequent in infants (116 pts.) than in older children (2762 pts.) with ALL in AIEOP series

	P value
WBC count $\geq 100 \times 10^3$/mmc	< .0001
Hepatosplenomegaly	< .0001
Failures to achieve CR	< .0001

Table 3. Progress of leukemic infants related for subtype of leukemia

	ALL		AnLL		Total	
	n	%	n	%	n	%
Registered	116		36		152	
too early to evaluate	5		1		6	
On study	111		35		146	
dead before any treatment	–		2		2	
Evaluable for CR	111	100	33	100	144	100
induction failure (death in IND)	23	19	10	7	33	26
CR	88	$\frac{79.3}{100}$	23	$\frac{69.7}{100}$	111	$\frac{77.1}{100}$
Death in CCR	8	9.1	2	8.7	10	9.0
Relapses	46		15		61	
BM	23		9		32	
CNS	15		1		16	
TES	2		1		3	
BM/CNS	3		1		4	
others combined	3		3		6	
Alive in CCR	34		6		40	

Early disease recurrence in this group, characterized by BM, CNS and testicular relapse (11 patients) and combined BM+CNS, BM+cutis, BM+test, BM+other (4 patients) (total: 15 patients, 65 %) was the major factor responsible for the poorest prognosis of this group of patients with AnLL.

Results

With a median follow-up time of 20 months, life table analysis conducted according to the Kaplan-Meier method showed a probability of overall survival (SUR) (95 % confidence limit) at 5 years of 30.2 % (40.3 - 20.1). As can be seen in figure 1, the product-limit estimate of SUR for infants with ALL is significantly different than that for children older than 1 year of age enrolled in AIEOP protocols during the study period ($p < .0001$).

The projected event-free survival (EFS) at 5 years for this group of infants is only 22.5 % (31.9 – 13.1) (fig. 2).

Initial WBC demonstrated a prognostic significance; in fact, event-free survival was significantly worse for infants with WBC in excess of $10 \times 10^3/$ mmc: 44.6 % vs 17.8 % (logrank p=0.033) (fig. 3).

In contrast to the situation observed in childhood ALL, the actuarial probability of event-free survival was not related to sex.

Moreover, the outcome of infants with ALL was not dependent on the specific therapeutic protocols in which the patients were entered, and no difference in terms of EFS were detected in infants <6 versus infants ≥6 months.

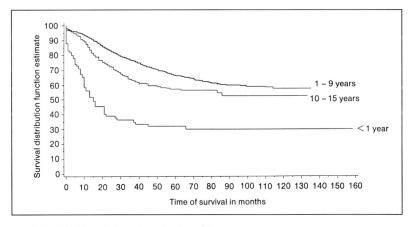

Fig. 1 AIEO/ALL in infants (survival by age).

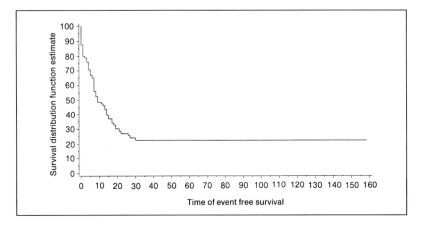

Fig. 2. AIEOP/ALL in fants (Event-free survival).

Although the number of long-term disease-free survivors is small, ten infants with ALL progressed in Continuous Complete Remission with a median follow-up of 4.5 years following cessation of therapy.

The actuarial EFS for the AnLL group was 20.5 % at 5 years. Only 5 infants with AnLL in 1st CR survived 6 years following cessation of therapy.

Discussion

Our data confirm that ALL patients of this age group have an increased incidence of biological and clinical characteristics associated with poor prognosis (WBC count, organomegaly), even if some particular aspects such as T leukemia, mediastinal mass and, in our experience, CNS involvement at diagnosis, are not frequently encountered.

Furthermore, we found an increased number of chromosomal aberrations (10 of 24 patients evaluable), most notably t(4,11).

We confirm that infants with ALL have a significantly worse prognosis than older children; in fact this group shows the poorest outcome of any age group, defined by age and WBC count as prognostic factors. The lower CR rate of our group of patients is related to the excessive toxicity of the treatment. This may be directly related to the fact that many patients were treated before that implementation of supportive therapy (antimicrobial, transfusional, etc.). Furthermore, infants are at increased risk of infectious complications due to the immaturity of their immune system.

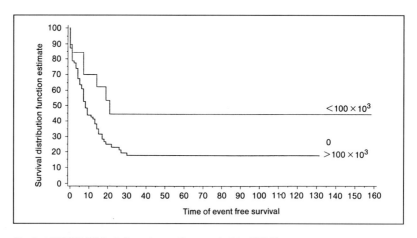

Fig. 3. AIEOP/ALL in infants (event free survival by WBC).

The early disease recurrence, most characterized by BM and CNS relapse, was the major fact responsible for the poor outcome of this patient group.

In AnLL, excess of FAB M4 and M5 morphology, and an increased rate of CNS leukemia at diagnosis can explain the poor response to therapy and outcome.

In conclusion, adverse biological-clinical aspects and response to therapy suggest that a new strategical approach of treatment such as new drugs or BM transplant must be investigated for this group of patients with acute leukemia. Leukemia in infants may be considered the most acute high-risk entity in need of a specialized treatment.

Summary

Data of 152 infants within cooperative trials (1975–1989) of the Italian Pediatric Hematology-Oncology Group are presented. 116 (76 %) had Acute Lymphoblastic Leukemia (ALL), 36 (24 %) had Acute Non-Lymphoblastic Leukemia (ANLL). Median initial white blood cell counts (WBC) were 64×10^3 pro μl for ALL, and 36×10^3 pro μl for ANLL. Leukemia karyotypes could be determined in 24 patients, and 10 abnormal ones were found, of which 4 had a chromosome translocation t(4;11). In the 34 patients with ANLL myelomonocytic (FAB-M_4) and monoblastic (FAB-M_5), cytomorphology prevailed. Overall survival probability at 5 years was 30 %, independent of specific therapeutic protocols. Initial WBC, however, was of prognostic significance.

References

1   Reaman G, Zeltzer P, Bleyer WA, et al: Acute lymphoblastic leukemia in infants less than one year of age: A cumulative experience of the children's cancer study group. J Clin Oncol 1985;3:1513–1521.
2   Crist WM, Pullen J, Boyett J, et al: Clinical and biological features predict a poor prognosis in acute lymphoid leukemias in infants: Pediatric Oncology Group Study. Blood 1986;67:135–140.
3   Pui CH, Raimondi SC, Murphy SB, et al: An analysis of leukemic cell chromosomal features in infants. Blood 1987;69:1289–1293.
4   Reaman GH: Special consideration for the infant with cancer, in Pizzo PA, Poplack DG (eds): Principles and practice of pediatric oncology. Philadelphia, Lippincott, 1989, pp 263–274.

Dr. Carlo Guazelli, IIIa. Clinica Pediatrica, Ematologia, Ospedale Meyer, Via Luca Giordano 13, I-50100 Firenze (Italy)

Contrib Oncol. Basel, Karger, 1990, vol 41, pp 18–29.

Acute Lymphoblastic Leukemia in Infants: Clinical Characteristics and Response to Therapy in the Multicenter Therapy Studies ALL-BFM 70/76/79/81/83/86

P. Bucsky [a], *S. Sauter* [a], *R. Dopfer* [b], *R. Gerein* [c], *J. Kühl* [d], *A. Reiter* [a], *J. Ritter* [e], *H. Riehm* [a]

[a] Department of Pediatrics, Medical School of Hannover
[b] Department of Pediatrics, University of Tübingen
[c] Department of Pediatrics, University of Frankfurt
[d] Department of Pediatrics, University of Würzburg
[e] Department of Pediatrics, University of Münster, FRG

Zusammenfassung

Die ALL hat eine schlechtere Prognose im Säuglingsalter (Leukämie-freies Überleben nur 26 %) im Vergleich zu höheren Altersstufen. Die Analyse von 6 BFM-Multizenterstudien an 71 Säuglingen (40 davon weniger als 6 Monate alt) zeigte, daß im Säuglingsalter prognostisch ungünstige Subtypen vorherrschen, die durch große Leukämiezellmasse, fehlende FAB-L1-Zellmorphologie, initiale ZNS-Leukämie, Kortikosteroid-Nichtansprechen, Therapietodesfälle und hohe Rezidivquote, besonders im ZNS, charakterisiert sind. Vor allem unter 6 Monate alte Säuglinge haben ein hohes Rückfallrisiko. In der zweiten Hälfte des Säuglingsalters scheint sich eine Verschiebung zu prognostisch besseren Typen anzubahnen. Spezielle Therapieprotokolle, möglichst auf internationaler Basis, für Säuglinge unter 6 Monate mit ALL, sind empfehlenswert.

Introduction

Childhood acute lymphoblastic leukemia (ALL) is clinically and biologically a heterogenous neoplastic disease. To predict the probability of continuous complete remission (pCCR), certain risk criteria were developed by retrospective analysis of clinical trials. These risk factors include clinical features as well as biological characteristics. Many of these risk criteria are closely associated, others are independent predictors of outcome despite risk-adapted therapy. Age and treatment regimen are such independent predictors of outcome in childhood ALL [1-3, 5-7, 14]. Virtually all therapy studies (including the BFM studies) demonstrate that infants have a less favorable prognosis than children of other age groups. In this report, we will retrospectively evaluate the clinical presentation at diagnosis and therapy response of infants treated according to six consecutive therapy studies of the BFM Study Group.

Material and Methods

71 children aged twelve months or less (≤ 12 months) at diagnosis were enrolled in the six consecutive multicenter therapy studies ALL-BFM 70,76,79,81,83, and the ongoing trial 86. Date of analysis was September 31, 1989. Of the 71 infants (2,7 % of the total study population), 40 children were in the age of six months or less (≤ 6 months) at diagnosis. For comparative analysis, we evaluated 69 children aged twelve to eighteen months ($>12-\leq 18$ months), 131 children aged eighteen to 24 months ($>18-\leq 24$ months), and 1734 patients aged two to ten years ($>2-\leq 10$ years) treated during the same study period (table 1). The morphological diagnosis of ALL was determined in bone marrow and peripheral blood smears stained by standard methods for Giemsa, periodic acid Schiff reagent, non-specific esterase and peroxidase. The protocol designs of the BFM Study Group have previously been reported [15-21]. The analysis was performed according to the recommendation of the 'Rome Workshop 85' [11]. For statistical evaluation and life table analysis, the methods of Cox, Kaplan and Meier were used [4, 8]. Immunological and cytogenetic data are not subjects of this analysis, and will be discussed separately.

Results

The probability of pCCR for the 71 infants was 0.26 at fourteen years (fig. 1). Clinically infant ALL was characterized by a very large tumor bur-

Table 1. Number of infants and children in the age groups evaluated in six consecutive therapy studies of the BFM Study Group

Age	No. of patients	in 1. CR	pCCR
$\leq$ 6 months	40	14	0.17
6 - $\leq$ 12 months	31	18	0.46
12 - $\leq$ 18 months	69	49	0.64
18 - $\leq$ 24 months	131	94	0.67
2 - $\leq$ 10 years	1734	1311	0.70

CR: complete remission; pCCR: probability of continuous complete remission.

den. Compared to other age groups, the initial blast count was very high in these children, especially in infants ≦6 months of age at diagnosis (table 2). The large tumor load was reflected in the high score for the 'BFM risk factor', which is based on blast cell count at diagnosis, liver size and spleen size [9]. There was a significant difference between the risk factors in the infant group compared to the group of children aged >2-≦10 years (p=0.001), and between patients aged ≦6 months compared to children aged >18-≦24 months at diagnosis (p=0.001; fig. 2).

Central nervous system (CNS) involvement at diagnosis is another important clinical feature. CNS disease at presentation was diagnosed in ten of 40

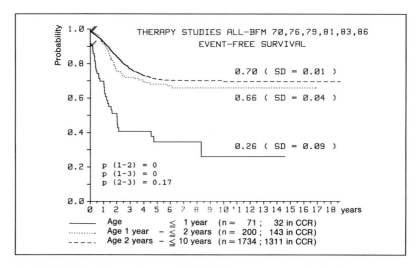

Fig. 1. Probability of event free survival for different age groups in the six consecutive ALL-BMF therapy studies.

Table 2. Median of the initial blast cell count in the different age groups

Age	Median*
≦ 6 months	196,700
6 - ≦ 12 months	43,800
12 - ≦ 18 months	11,700
18 - ≦ 24 months	6,700
2 - ≦ 10 years	4,000

* median of initial blast cell count / μl.

patients (25 %) in the age group ≦6 months, six of 31 patients (19 %) aged
>6-≦12 months and four of 69 patients (6 %) aged >12-≦18 months at diag-
nosis. There was a significant difference in the incidence of initial CNS involvement in the group of infants ≦6 months of age compared to the group of
patients who were in age of >12-≦18 months at diagnosis (p=0.001; tables 3, 4).

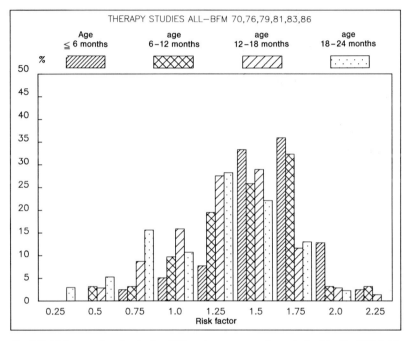

Fig. 2. Initial tumor burden in the different age groups characterized by the BFM risk
factor. See also text.

Table 3. CNS involvement at the time of diagnosis and initial blast cell count in the age
groups

Age	No. of patients					
	* CNS	in 1. CR	>100,000	>50,000/μl	Total	in 1. CR
≦ 6 months	10	2	28	29	40	14
6 - ≦ 12 months	6	2	13	18	31	18
12 - ≦ 18 months	4	3	11	20	69	49

*CNS: leukemic involvement of central nervous system at diagnosis; CR: complete remission.

In studies ALL-BFM 83 and 86, fifteen of the 43 patients (35 %) aged ≦12 months and six of 36 patients (16 %) aged >12 -≦18 months failed to respond to the initial corticosteroid therapy [20]. In study ALL-BFM 86, fifteen patients aged ≦12 months (nine infants aged ≦6 months and six in age >6 -≦12 months) were classified in the high risk patient group 'EG' (table 5). In a recently published study [7], sex was considered to be an independent prognostic variable, having low degrees of association or interaction to other factors favoring female patients. However, in the infant patient population it cannot be confirmed. Moreover, a slight but not significant advantage for boys in outcome can be stated in the BFM studies (table 6).

The prognostic significance of blast cell morphology according to the FAB classification has been well documented in many studies. In therapy study ALL-BFM 86, less favorable FAB-subtypes occur more often in very young patients: Nine of 19 infants aged ≦6 months presented a non-FAB-L1 blast cell morphology at diagnosis.

Table 4. Correlation between age, initial CNS involvement and initial blast cell count

Initial blast cell count CNS disease at diagnosis	<50,000/μl		>=50,000/μl	
	+	−	+	−
Age	No. of patients			
≦ 6 months	1	10	9	20
6 - ≦ 12 months	2	11	4	15
12 - ≦ 18 months	2	46	2	19

CNS: central nervous system.

Table 5. Number of high risk patients (EG) and prednisolon poor responders in the different age groups in the ongoing trial. In these patients protocol E of the study ALL-BFM 86 was applied

Age	No. of patients				
	P-PR	EG	in 1. CR	Total	in 1. CR
≦ 6 months	9	9	4	19	10
6 - ≦ 12 months	4	6	6	9	8
12 - ≦ 18 months	2	5	5	15	14

P-PR: prednisolon poor-responder; EG: high risk patient group for protocol E; CR: complete remission.

Concerning the response to treatment, there was no significant difference in the complete remission (CR) rate for infants compared to other age groups: The CR rate was 89 % for children aged ≦6 months, compared to 98 % for patients in age >2−≦10 years at diagnosis. Early failures by non-response seem to influence the therapy results only in the infant group aged ≦6 months: Four of 40 infants did not respond to therapy. These early failures were partially responsible for the initial outdrop in this age group. Death secondary to therapy related toxicity occurred in ten of the 71 infants, but in none of the patients aged >12−≦18 months at diagnosis (table 7).

The probability of recurrence of leukemia was 38 % in infants aged ≦12 months (table 8). In contrast, patients aged >2−≦10 years had a relative risk of relapse of only 20 %. The probability of CNS relapse or involvement of CNS in relapse was 25 % in the infant group aged ≦6 months, compared to the 14 % in the group of patients aged >2−≦10 years (p=0.03).

Table 6. In the infant patient groups a slight but not significant difference in pCCR could be observed, favoring male patients

Age	No. of patients		pCCR		SD	
	f	m	f	m	f	m
≦ 6 months	19	21	0.14	0.22	0.12	0.11
6 − ≦ 12 months	14	17	0.39	0.56	0.16	0.13
12 − ≦ 18 months	26	43	0.74	0.60	0.10	0.09

pCCR: probability of continuous complete remission; SD: standard deviation; f: female; m: male.

Table 7. Patients died due to ALL as non-responder or to therapy related toxicity / in complete remission

Age	No. of patients	Ceased			
		ALL	NR	Therapy	in CR
≦ 6 months	40	10	4	6	2
6 − ≦ 12 months	31	3	–	4	1
12 − ≦ 18 months	69	5	–	–	–

NR: non-responder; CR: complete remission.

As to the clinical outcome, children in age ≦6 months at diagnosis had a pCCR of 0.17, compared to 0.46 in children aged >6-≦12 months (fig. 3). During the study periods, the prognosis for infants could be improved. The pCCR was 0.26 for the total study population (fig. 1), compared to 0.36 for infants treated on studies ALL-BFM 81, 83, and 86 (fig. 4). However, this improvement was not observed in the infant group aged ≦6 months: The pCCR was 0.17 for all studies (fig. 3), compared to 0.18 in the three more recent therapy studies (fig. 5). Comparing the pCCR for infants with an initial blast cell count <50,000/ul versus >50,000/ul in the age group ≦6

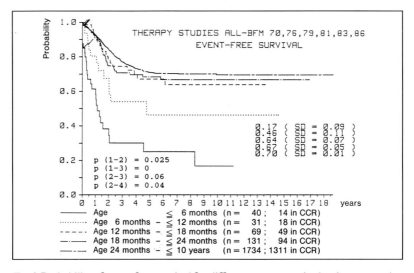

Fig. 3. Probability of event free survival for different age groups in the six consecutive ALL-BFM therapy studies.

Table 8. Localization of relapses in the different age groups

Age	No. of patients	BM	CNS	Testis	BM + CNS	BM + Testis	*	total
≦ 6 months	40	9	3	1	1	0	1	15
6 - ≦ 12 months	31	3	4	0	1	2	0	10
12 - ≦ 18 months	69	4	6	1	6	1	0	18

BM: bone marrow; CNS: central nervous system; mo: months; *: other localisation of relapse.

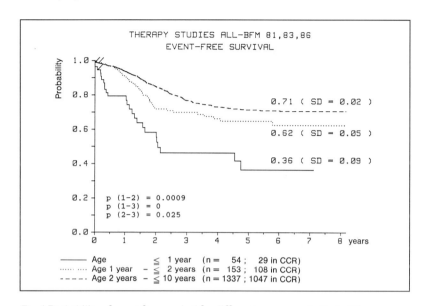

Fig. 4. Probability of event free survival for different age groups in the last three consecutive ALL-BFM therapy studies.

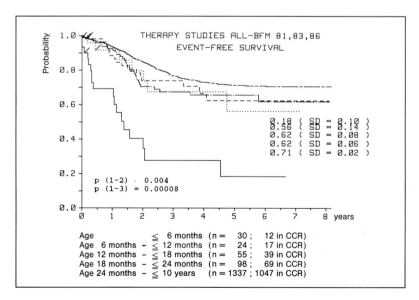

Fig. 5. Probability of event free survival for different age groups in the last three consecutive ALL-BFM therapy studies.

months, no difference in pCCR could be observed (fig. 6). In addition, in the six consecutive multicenter therapy studies of the BFM Study Group, only one patient could be diagnosed within the first 28 days of life. In a new-born, ALL was present on day nine after birth. A complete remission could be achieved and now maintenance therapy is applied.

Discussion

Similar to other studies [1, 2, 6, 7, 13, 14], this clinical evaluation confirms the unfavorable prognosis of ALL in infants. The poor outcome is reflected by certain clinical features at diagnosis. In particular, a very high tumor load can be observed, especially in patients ≦6 months of age. Another unfavorable clinical feature is the high incidence of CNS involvement at diagnosis and in relapse. There was a strong correlation between initial blast cell count and CNS disease at diagnosis with age: The youngest patients had the highest initial blast cell count and/or the highest frequency of CNS involvement at the time of diagnosis. The negative clinical features of high tumor burden, high incidence of CNS involvement, poor cortico-steroid response, and high risk of relapse may reflect the particular clinical

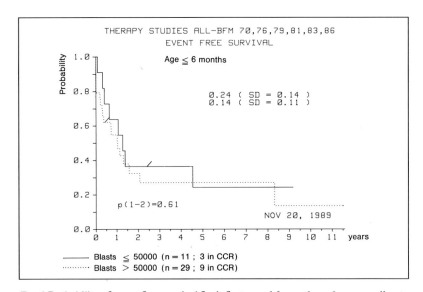

Fig. 6. Probability of event free survival for infants aged 6 months or less according to the inital blast cell count in the six consecutive ALL-BFM therapy studies.

characteristics of infant leukemia. In addition, the significance of age ≦6 months as an independent prognostic factor could be observed. Concerning the biology of the leukemic blast cells, specific cytogenetic aberrations, and certain immunological subtypes of ALL have been described in infant patients. Chromosomal regions preferentially involved in infant leukemia include 11q23–25, 9p21–22 and 10p11–13 [12]. CD10 (cALLa)-negative 0-ALL, CD10- and Tdt-negative acute undifferentiated leukemia occur more often in the infant populations [1, 10]. All these biological characteristics of blast cells are most likely reflected in the peculiar clinical features and poor outcome of ALL in infancy. However, in this respect the particular biology of infants by itself may play an important role, as well. A change of clinical characteristics to prognostically more favorable subtypes of ALL seems to occur during the second half of the first year of life. Our evaluations suggest that new therapy regimens are needed for therapy of infant leukemia, particularly for infants aged ≦6 months at diagnosis. These new regimens should be more specific, thus more effective for this rather distinguished subgroup of childhood ALL, at the same, time life-threatening toxicity, especially during the induction phase of treatment, has to be avoided.

In summary, this analysis illustrates that clinically less favorable subtypes of ALL are more common in infancy, thus explaining at least partially the impaired outcome. These subtypes are characterized by very large tumor load with non-FAB-L1 morphology, CNS disease at diagnosis, corticosteroid poor-response, frequent failures by non-response, and death due to therapy toxicity and high relapse rate, particularly in CNS. Infants ≦6 months of age are at especially high risk. Age ≦6 months seems to be an independent prognostic variable. A change of clinical features to prognostically more favorable subtypes of ALL occurs in the second half of the first year of life. For further unterstanding of the biology of ALL in this rather peculiar patient subset, an international therapy study for infants would be helpful.

Summary

Age and treatment are important prognostic factors of treatment outcome in childhood ALL. Infant patients have, in contrast to all other age groups, a less favorable prognosis (leukemia-free survival only 26 %). The analysis of six multicenter therapy studies of the BFM Study Group with 71 infants (40 less than 6 months of age) illustrates that clinically less favorable subtypes of ALL are more common in infancy, thus explaining at least partially the impaired outcome. These subtypes are characterized by very large tumor burden with non-FAB-L1 morphology, CNS disease at diagnosis, poor response corticosteroids, frequent failures by non-response and death due to therapy toxicity, and high relapse rate, particularly in CNS. Infants ≤ 6 months of age are at especially high risk. Age ≤ 6 months seems to be an independent prognostic variable, having low degrees of association or interaction. A change of clinical features to prognostically more favorable subtypes in ALL occurs in the second half of the first year of life. This evaluation suggests that for therapy of infant ALL, particularly for infants aged six months or less, a more specific and thus more effective treatment regimen is needed. For further understanding of the biology of ALL in this rather peculiar patient subset, an international therapy study for infants would be helpful.

References

1   Bucsky P, Brämswig JH, Dopfer R, Gerein V, Kühl J, Neidhardt MK, Riehm H: Acute lymphoblastic leukemia of infancy: Phenotypes and prognosis in three BFM trials. 4th Int. Symposion on Therapy of Acute Leukemias. Rome, 1987; Feb. 7-12, Abstracts p 166.

2   Bucsky P, Reiter A, Ritter J, Dopfer R, Riehm H: Die akute lymphoblastische Leukämie im Säuglingsalter: Ergebnisse aus fünf multizentrischen Therapiestudien ALL-BFM 1970-1986. Klin Pädiatr 1988;200:177-183.

3   Camitta B, Crist W, Pullen J, Boyett J, Frankel L: Acute lymphoblastic leukemia (ALL) in infants: Clinical and biological features predict poor response to therapy. 4th Int. Symposion on Therapy of Acute Leukemias. Rome, 1987: Feb. 7-12, Abstracts p 166.

4   Cox DR: Regression models and life tables. J Roy Stat Soc Bull 1972;34:187-220.

5   Christ W, Boyett J, Pullen J, van Eys J, Vietti T: Clinical and biological features predict poor prognosis in acute lymphoid leukemias in children and adolescents: A Pediatric Oncology Group review. Med Pediat Oncol 1986;14:135-140.

6   Christ W, Pullen J, Boyett J, Falletta J, van Eys J, Borowitz M, Jackson J, Dowell B, Frankel L, Quddus F, Ragab A, Vietti T: Clinical and biological features predict a poor prognosis in acute lymphoid leukemia in infants: A Pediatric Oncology Group Study. Blood 1986;67:135-140.

7   Hammond D, Sather H, Nesbit M, Miller D, Coccia P, Bleyer A, Lukens J, Siegel S: Analysis of prognostic factors in acute lymphoblastic leukemia. Med Pediat Oncol 1986;14:124-134.

8   Kaplan EL, Meier P: Nonparametric estimation from incomplete observations. J Am Stat Ass 1958;53:457-481.

9   Langermann HJ, Henze G, Wulf M, Riehm H: Abschätzung der Tumorzellmasse bei der akuten lymphoblastischen Leukämie im Kindesalter: Prognostische Bedeutung und praktische Anwendung. Klin Pädiat 1982;194:209-213.

10 Ludwig WD, Bartram CR, Harbott J, Köller U, Haas OA, Hansen-Hagge T, Heil G, Seibt-Jung H, Teichmann JV, Ritter J, Knapp W, Gadner H, Thiel E, Riehm H: Phenotypic and genotypic heterogeneity in infant acute leukemia I. Acute lymphoblastic leukemia. Leuk 1989;3:431-439.

11   Mastrangelo R, Poplack D, Bleyer A, Riccardi R, Sather H, D'Angio G: Report and recommendations of the Rome Workshop concerning poor-prognosis acute lymphoblastic leukemia in children: Biological bases for staging, stratification, and treatment. Med Pediat Oncol 1986;14:191–194.

12   Pui CH, Raimondi CR, Murphy SB, Ribeiro RC, Kalwinsky DK, Dahl GV, Christ WM, Williams DL: An analysis of leukemic cell chromosomal feature in infants. Blood 1987;69:1289–1293.

13   Reaman GH, Zeltzer P, Bleyer WA, Amendola B, Level C, Sather H, Hammond GD: Acute lymphoblastic leukemia (ALL) in infants less than one year of age. A cumulative experience of the Children's Cancer Study Group (CCSG). Proc Am Soc Clin Oncol 1983;2:C–321.

14   Reaman GH, Zeltzer P, Bleyer WA, Amendola B, Level C, Sather H, Hammond GD: Acute lymphoblastic leukemia in infants less then one year of age: A cumulative experience of the Childrens Cancer Study Group. J Clin Oncol 1985;3:1513–1521.

15   Riehm H, Feickert HJ, Lampert F: Acute lymphoblastic leukemia, in Voute PA, Barrett A, Bloom HJG, Lemerle J, Neidhardt MK: (eds): Cancer in children. Berlin, Springer, 1986, pp 101–118.

16   Riehm H, Feickert HJ, Schrappe M, Henze G, Schellong G: Therapy results in five ALL-BFM studies since 1970: Implications of risk factors for prognosis. Haematol Blood Transfus 1981;30:139–146.

17   Riehm H, Gadner H, Henze G, Kornhuber B, Langermann HJ, Müller-Weihrich S, Schellong G: Acute lymphoblastic leukemia: treatment results in three BFM studies (1979–1981), in Murphy SB, Gilbert JR (eds): Leukemia research: Advances in cell biology and treatment. Amsterdam, Elsevier, 1983, pp 251–263.

18   Riehm H, Gadner H, Henze G, Langermann HJ, Odenwald E: The Berlin childhood acute lymphoblastic leukemia therapy study, 1970–76. Am J Pediat Hematol Oncol, 1980;2:299–306.

19   Riehm H, Gadner H, Welte K: Die West-Berliner Studie zur Behandlung der akuten lymphoblastischen Leukämie des Kindes – Erfahrungsbericht nach 6 Jahren. Klin Pädiat 1977;189:89–101.

20   Riehm H, Reiter A, Schrappe M, Berthold F, Dopfer R, Gerein V, Ludwig R, Ritter J, Stollmann B, Henze G: Die Corticosteroid-abhängige Dezimierung der Leukämiezellzahl im Blut als Prognosefaktor bei der akuten lymphoblastischen Leukämie im Kindesalter (Therapiestudie ALL-BFM 83). Klin Pädiat 1986;199:151–160.

21   Schrappe M, Beck J, Brandeis WE, Feickert HJ, Gadner H, Graf N, Havers W, Henze G, Jobke A, Kornhuber B, Kühl J, Lampert F, Müller-Weirich S, Niethammer D, Reiter A, Rister M, Ritter J, Schellong G, Tausch W, Weinel P, Riehm H: Die Behandlung der akuten lymphoblastischen Leukämie im Kindes- und Jugendalter: Ergebnisse der multizentrischen Therapiestudie ALL-BFM 81. Klin Pädiat 1987;199:133–150.

Dr. Peter Bucsky, Kinderklinik der MHH,
Postfach 61 01 80, Konstanty-Gutschow-Str. 8, D-3000 Hannover (FRG)

Contrib Oncol. Basel, Karger, 1990, vol 41, pp 30–35.

Acute Myelogenous Leukemia in the First Year of Life

Analysis and Treatment Results of 25 Infants of the German Cooperative Studies AML-BFM 78 and 83 [1]

J. Ritter[a], *U. Creutzig*[a], *A. Jobke*[b], *F. Lampert*[c], *A. Reiter*[d], *G. Schellong*[a]

[a] Children's Hospital, University of Münster
[b] Children's Hospital, University of Freiburg
[c] Children's Hospital, University of Gießen
[d] Cnopf'sche Kinderklinik, Nürnberg, FRG

Zusammenfassung

25 der 333 Kinder (7,5 %), welche in die beiden multizentrischen Therapiestudien AML-BMF-78 und -83 zwischen Dezember 1978 und Oktober 1986 aufgenommen wurden, befanden sich zum Zeitpunkt der Diagnose im Säuglingsalter. Es bestanden keine signifikanten Unterschiede hinsichtlich der Geschlechtsverteilung oder der Häufigkeit eines initialen ZNS-Befalls. Akute Monoblastenleukämien (FAB M5) fanden sich signifikant häufiger bei Säuglingen (12/25, 48 %) als bei älteren Kindern (22 %). Die Behandlungsergebnisse bei Säuglingen und älteren Kindern unterschieden sich nicht signifikant: 75 % der Säuglinge und 80 % der älteren Kinder erreichten eine komplette Remission. Die Lifetable-Analyse ergab eine nahezu identische Wahrscheinlichkeit des ereignisfreien Überlebens nach 8 Jahren bei Säuglingen (pCCR = 40 %; SD = 10 %) und älteren Kindern (pCCR = 43 %; SD = 3 %). Zusammenfassend bestehen Unterschiede bei der klinischen Präsentation zwischen Säuglingen und älteren Kindern mit AML. Unter den Bedingungen der AML-Studie BFM-78 und BFM-83 bestehen jedoch keine Unterschiede im Behandlungsergebnis zwischen Säuglingen und älteren Kindern.

Introduction

Acute myelogenous leukemia (AML) during the first year of life is a rare event. Diagnosis and treatment of the infants with AML pose many difficult challenges to the multidisciplinary pediatric oncologic team. Espe-

[1] Supported by the Bundesministerium für Forschung und Technologie, FRG

cially the increased toxicity of some cytotoxic drugs and special problems in supportive care have to be considered in this age group.

However, published data on the prognosis of infant leukemia do not provide conclusive results whether the outcome in this age group is different in comparison to older children. Therefore, we analysed the initial patient characteristics and the treatment outcome of infants and older children which entered the two German multicenter studies AML-BFM 78 and 83.

Patients and Methods

Ten out of 151 children in study-AML-BFM 78 and 15 out of 182 children in study AML-BFM 83 were less than 12 months of age at diagnosis. Definitions of AML and reasons for exclusion from the study were identical in infants and older children [1, 2, 6]. Therapy was identical for infants and older children [2, 8]. However, it was recommended in both studies to calculate the dosage of cytotoxic drugs according to kilograms of body weight in children weighing less than 10 kg instead of calculating dosages according to square meter of body surface, which is recommended for children weighing more than 10 kg. The recommended dose for cranial irradiation was 12 Gy for children less than 12 months of age, 15 Gy for children between 12 and 24 months of age, and 18 Gy for older children. The recommended dosage for intrathecal chemotherapy was age-adjusted.

Kaplan-Meyer life-table-analyses were based on the following definitions:

Event-free-survival (EFS): In the whole group of patients all events leading to remission failures (early death, non-response) or termination of first remission (relapse, death during complete remission) were evaluated.

All children who died during the first 6 weeks after starting treatment were defined as early death patients. Children who died before the onset of therapy were not included in the life-table-analysis.

Follow-up data were actualized as of March 1, 1989.

Results

Twenty-five (7,5 %) of 333 children entering the two studies were less than 1 year of age at diagnosis. Table 1 shows some patient characteristics of these 25 infants as compared to the 308 older children. There was no significant difference in sex distribution, median WBC or incidence of CNS involvement at diagnosis.

In table 2, some prognostically important morphological characteristics of the leukemic blasts are shown for both age groups, such as the morphological subtype according to the FAB classification [1], presence of Auer rods [7], and presence of eosinophilia of ≥ 3 % within the bone marrow [8].

The prevalence of acute monoblastic leukemia (FAB M5) was significantly (p<0.01) higher in infants (12/25; 48 %) than in older children (22 %). The differentiated granulocytic subtypes FAB M2 and M3 were not seen in infants, in contrast to older children (26.5 %). The prevalence of AML with Auer rods and AML with bone marrow eosinophilia (≥3 %) was significantly (p<0.05) lower in infants. The overall treatment results of infants and older children of both studies are given in table 3. The CR rate was 75 % in infants and 80 % in older children (p=n.s.). After a median follow-up time of more than 8 years, a relapse occurred in 8/18 infants (44 %) and in 39 % of the older children (p=n.s.).

Significantly (p<0.05) more relapses with involvement of extramedullary sites occurred in infants (5/8) than in older children (19/93). Relapses with CNS involvement occurred in 3 of the 8 relapsing infants as compared to 13 of 93 relapsing older children. These 3 infants with relapses involving the CNS did not receive CNS directed therapy because of the very young age of less than 6 months of diagnosis. Two infants with later relapses involving the CNS suffered from AMOL (FAB M5) and the third from AMML (FAB M4).

Table 1. Patient characteristics – AML BFM 78 and 83

	< 1 yr	> 1 yr
n	25	308
male	15 (63 %)	165 (53,5 %)
CNS [+] at Dx	2 (8 %)	15 (5 %)
WBC >100,000/μl	8 (32 %)	72 (23 %)

Table 2. Morphological characteristics – AML BFM 78 and 83

	< 1 yr	> 1 yr	p
FAB M1	4 (16 %)	69 (23 %)	n.s.
M2	0	71 (23 %)	–
M3	0	11 (3,5 %)	–
M4	7 (28 %)	78 (25 %)	n.s.
M5	12 (48 %)	68 (22 %)	< 0.01
M6	2 (8 %)	8 (2,5 %)	
M7	0	3 (1 %)	
Auer rods	2 / 20 (10 %)	135 / 263 (51 %)	< 0.01
Eos. ≥ 3 % (BM)	2 / 20 (10 %)	73 / 251 (29 %)	< 0.05

Life-table analysis revealed a nearly identical probability of event-free-survival after 8 years in infants (pCCR=40 %; SD=10 %) and older children (pCCR=43 %; SD=3 %, fig. 1). In both studies, about 50 % (3/7 in study BFM-78 and 6/11 in study BFM-83) of all infants coming into remission are alive and without evidence of disease after a median follow-up time of more than 9 years in study BFM-78 and 5 years in study BFM-83.

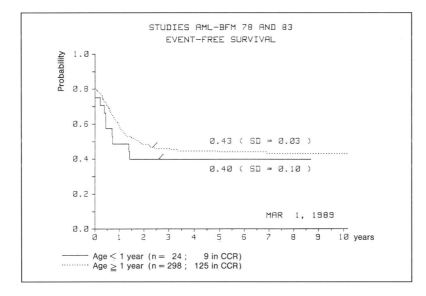

Fig. 1. Probability of event-free survival after 8 years in infants and older children of studies AML-BFM 78 and 83

Table 3. Treatment results – AML BFM 78 and 83

	< 1 yr	> 1 yr	p
n	25	308	
Death before therapy	1 (4 %)	10 (3 %)	n.s.
Early death	4 (16 %)	25 (8 %)	n.s.
Non-responder	2 (8 %)	33 (11 %)	n.s.
CR	18 (75 %)	240 (80 %)	n.s.
Relapses	8 (44 %)	93 (31 %)	n.s.
Death in 1. CR	0	10	
Lost to follow-up	1	12	
(BMT in 1. CR)	0	9	
In 1 CCR	9 (50 %)	125 (52 %)	n.s.

Discussion

The prevalence of AML in the first year of life was comparable in both German multicenter AML-BFM studies. Altogether 25/333 children (7.5 %) were less than one year of age at diagnosis. As others described in infant AUL/ALL [5], we found some biological differences between infant AML and AML in older children. The prevalence of acute monoblastic leukemia (FAB M5) was significantly higher in infants than in older children. Nearly half (12 of 25) of the infants described in this study suffered from acute monoblastic leukemia. On the other hand, the differentiated granulocytic subtypes FAB M2 and M3 did not occur in infants in the present study. About one third of the infants had hyperleukocytosis (WBC $\geq 100,000/\mu l$), as compared to 23 %. Similar results were described by other multicenter studies of childhood AML. In a recent CCSG study, hyperleukocytosis, CNS leukemia at diagnosis and skin infiltration were found to occur significantly more often in infants than in older children with AML [3]. The VAPA study from Boston described an excess of the FAB subtypes M4 and M5 in infant AML, which was associated with a less favorable prognosis [9].

The outcome for infants with AML in the present study was not significantly different than that for older children. This was true both for remission induction and for remission duration. These findings confirm data from the CCSG [3], which also described no differences in either complete remission rate or survival at three years between infants and older children. However, the rate of 50 % long-term survivors of infants in the present study is superior to the rate of 20 % long-term survivors in the CCSG study, reflecting the overall better outcome of the AML-BFM studies in comparison to other published chemotherapy studies for childhood AML [4].

Because of the relatively low number of infants with AML in the present study, no detailed risk factor analysis was done within this small group of patients. Risk factor analysis of the whole group of children with AML entering the BFM studies revealed that the FAB subtype M5 is a risk factor for relapse under the conditions of study AML-BFM 83 [8].

Summary

25 of 333 children (7.5 %) who entered the two German multicenter studies AML-BFM-78 and -83 between December 1978 and October 1986 were under one year of age at

diagnosis. There were no differences as to sex distribution, median WBC or incidence of initial CNS involvement between these 25 infants and the 308 older children. The prevalence of acute monoblastic leukemia (FAB M5) was significantly higher in infants (12/25; 48 %) than in the older children (22 %). Overall treatment results were not significantly different between infants and older children: The rate of complete remission was 75 % in infants vs. 80 % in older children. Kaplan-Meier estimates for the event-free-survival after 8 years revealed nearly identical results in infants (pCCR = 40 %; SD = 10 %) and older children (pCCR = 43 %; SD = 3 %). In conclusion, although there are some biological differences between infants and older children with AML, the treatment outcome for infants with AML is not significantly different from that of older children under the conditions of the AML studies BFM-78 and -83.

References

1   Bennett JM, Catovsky D, Daniel MT, Flandrin G, Dalton DAG, Gralnick HR, Sultan C: Proposals for the classification of the acute leukaemias. Br J Haemato 1976;33:451.
2   Creutzig U, Ritter J, Riehm H, Langermann HJ, Henze G, Kabisch H, Niethammer D, Jürgens H, Stollmann B, Lasson U, Kaufmann U, Löffler H, Schellong G: Improved treatment results in childhood acute myelogenous leukemia: A report of the German Cooperative Study AML-BFM 78. Blood 1985;65:298.
3   Lampkin B, Buckley J, Nesbit N et al: Clinical and laboratory findings and response to therapy in infants less than one year of age with acute non-lymphocytic leukemia (ANLL) Proc Am Soc Clin Oncol 1984;3:785.
4   Lie SO: Acute myelogenous leukaemia in children. Eur J Pediat 1989;148:382.
5   Reaman G, Zeltzer P, Bleyer WA et al: Acute lymphoblastic leukemia in infants less than one year of age. A culmulative experience at the Children's Cancer Study Group. J Clin Oncol 1985;3:1513–1521.
6   Ritter J, Creutzig U, Riehm HJ, Schellong G: Acute myelogenous leukemia: current status of therapy in children. Recent Res Cancer Res 1984;93:204–215.
7   Ritter J, Creutzig U, Schellong G: Prognostic significance of Auer rods in childhood AML: results of the studies AML-BFM 78 and 83. Med Pediat Oncol 1989;17:202–209.
8   Ritter J, Creutzig U, Schellong G: Improved treatment results in the myelocytic subtypes FAB M1–M4 but not in FAB M5 after intensification of induction therapy: results of the German childhood AML Studies BFM 78 and BFM 83 in Büchner T, Schellong G, Hiddemann W, Ritter J (eds): Acute Leukemias II. Haematol Blood Transfus. Berlin, Springer 1990, vol 33, pp 157–162.
9   Weinstein HJ, Mayer RJ, Rosenthal DS et al: Chemotherapy for acute myelogenous leukemia in children and adults. VAPA update. Blood 1983;62:315–319.

Prof. Dr. Jörg Ritter, Universitäts-Kinderklinik,
Albert-Schweitzer-Str. 33, D-4400 Münster (FRG)

Contrib Oncol. Basel, Karger, 1990, vol 41, pp 36–45.

The Immunophenotypic Analysis of Acute Non-Myeloid Leukemias in Infants
AIEOP Cooperative Study[1]

G. Basso, M. C. Putti, A. Cantù-Rajnoldi, M. Saitta, A. Comelli, M. Nardi, L. Nespoli, P. Paolucci, G. Russo, P. Biddau, T. Santostasi, N. Santoro, A. M. Lippi, L. Felici, R. Rondelli

Centro per la studio e la cura della leucemia infantile, Department of Pediatrics, University of Padua, Italy

Zusammenfassung

Akute Leukämie (AL) bei Säuglingen (unter 12 Monate alt) ist selten und hat oft besondere klinische (hohe Leukozytenzahl, Organomegalie) und zellbiologische (besonders zytogenetische) Eigenschaften. In dieser Arbeit werden die zellulären Immunophenotypen von 48 Fällen, die an verschiedenen italienischen Zentren behandelt wurden, analysiert. Nur 2 der Patienten hatten eine T-ALL. Alle anderen waren HLA-DR+, die Hälfte (23 Fälle) zeigten CD 10– Positivität. Hinweise für deren Zugehörigkeit zur B-Zell-Reihe waren CD19–, CD24– und TdT-Positivität, auch oft CD20+ und/oder CyIgM+ (reifer B-Zell Phenotyp). Die 23 CD10-negativen Fälle waren häufig positiv für TdT und CD19, aber meist negativ für CD24, CD20, CyIgM. Die Koexpression myeloischer Antigene auf CD10-negativen Leukämiezellen weist auf die Herkunft von einer primitiveren Zelle hin und berechtigt zur Definition «hybrid» AL. Weiterhin fanden sich besondere «hybride» chromosomale Translokationen wie die t(4;11) in den Leukämiezellen von 7 der CD10 negativen Fälle.

Introduction

In modern chemotherapeutic protocols of childhood acute lymphoblastic leukemias (ALL), the role of immunological phenotype in prognosis is under discussion. In fact, while in the late 70's the presence of E rosette or surface immunoglobulins were considered signs of severe prognosis, now,

[1] Supported by AIRC, ref.n.1412/88, by M.P.I. and by C.N.R., Progetto Finalizzato Oncologia

probably due to the good results obtained by more aggressive chemothera-
pies, the clinical features are the only important prognostic criteria [3, 4, 17].

The majority of children diagnosed with ALL can expect to experience
a long event-free survival; more than 60 % of these patients are in complete
remission after 4 years from diagnosis [14].

These good results have no value for infants, mostly because with
them the conventional anti-leukemic protocols are not efficient. Various
factors are probably involved in this poor response: The frequent high
white blood cell count and organomegaly, and also the presence of a high
percentage of specific cytogenetic abnormalities [6, 15, 19].

We examined in this study the immunological phenotype of 48 infants
younger than 12 months of age, referred from various Italian institutions
pertaining to the Italian Association of Hematology and Oncology
(AIEOP), in order to determine if the Italian patients have the same characteristics previously described in other series [5, 7, 12, 19], i.e., a low percentage of C-ALL antigen and a high frequency of coexpression of some myeloid antigens. Furthermore, we studied if the immunological markers could
identify different forms of acute leukemias in infants, hence utilizing different therapeutic regimens to improve the clinical response.

Materials and Methods

The immunological phenotypes of acute leukemia in 48 infants (age less than 12
months) of various AIEOP institutions were studied. The morphological and cytochemical
criteria utilized to enroll the patients in this study were those necessary to exclude the
diagnosis of acute myeloid leukemia, according to the FAB classification: Less than 3 % of
myeloperoxidase positivity and non-specific esterase negativity on blasts [2]. Moreover,
only the phenotypes studied by an adequate number of antibodies for a correct immunological diagnosis were included.

We examined monoclonal antibodies (moab) capable of identifying differentiation
antigens of B cells pertaining to CD19, CD24, CD20, CD10 and antigens of T cells belonging to CD1a, CD3, CD5, CD7 (table 1). To identify myeloid antigens, we utilized various
moab; some of them are clustered in CD11b, CD13, CD14, CD15, CD33, CDW65 and others, as NHL30.5, are not clustered.

Furthermore, surface (SmIg) and cytoplasmatic immunoglobulins (CyIgM) and
HLA-DR were investigated. All markers were studied by indirect immunofluorescence on
microscopy or flow cytometry. Moreover, the indirect immunofluorescence test with the
policlonal antibody for the detection of TdT (BRL) was performed on slides or cytospins. A
percentage of more than 20 % for each monoclonal antibody and of 10 % for CyIgM and
TdT was considered as positive.

Results

The immunological markers identified three principal groups. The first was composed of two cases (4 % of all patients) classified as T-ALL for CD7 and TdT positivity. In these cases the HLA-DR and the other B antigens studied were negative, except for CD10 positivity in one of them (table 2a).

The other 46 patients were divided into two groups on the basis of CD10 positivity or negativity. Some immunological markers were common to both groups, while for others the results were clearly different. In fact, all 46 A.L. demonstrated positivity regarding HLA-DR, and no relevant differences were found between the two groups in relation to CD19, CD9 and

Table 1. Immunological Reagents used for Phenotyping

CD/Ag	Antibody	Main cellular distribution	Source
B Cell Markers			
CD19	B4	pan B	Coulter
CD24	OKB2	pan B, PMNs	Ortho
CD9	BA2	pan B, Monocytes, pts	Hybritec
CD10	J5	early B, C-ALL	Coulter
CD20	B1	pan mature B	Coulter
- -	OKDR	HLA-DR	Ortho
SmIg	IgG, A, M	mature B	B.R.B.
CyIg	μ	pre-B	S.B.A.
T Cell Markers			
CD7	Leu9	panT	B.D.
CD1a	T6	thymocytes	Coulter
CD5	T1	panT	Coulter
CD3	Leu4	T cells	B.D.
Myeloid Markers			
CD11b	OKM1	granul./monocytes	Ortho
CD13	My7	granul./monocytes	Coulter
CD14	My4	monocytes	Coulter
CD15	LeuM1	granulocytes/PMNs	B.D.
CD33	My9	pan-myeloid	Coulter
CDW65	VIM2	granul./monocytes	B.R.B

Other antimyeloid MoAb not clustered were obtained from the II and III International Workshops [1].
B.D. Becton Dickinson
S.B.A. Southern Biotechnology Associated
B.R.B. Boehringer Robin Biochemia

TdT positivity. In the CD10+ group the percentage of CD19+ A.L. was 85%, as against 75% in the CD10− group. For CD9 and TdT the percentages were respectively 81% as against 85%, and 76% as against 70% (tables 2b, 2c).

In examining the CD 24, CD 20 and cytoplasmatic immunoglobulins, an important difference was evident. The CD24 antibody was positive in almost all C-ALL+ A.L. examined (96%), only one case being negative.

In this group one or both markers of more differentiated B cells (CD20 and CyIgM) were demonstrated in high percentage (61%, 14/23). These two markers were frequently simultaneously positive, but occasionaly CD20 was positive with absent CyIgM, and vice versa.

The classical C-ALL phenotype (TdT, CD19, CD24, CD10, HLA-DR) corresponding to the III stage of Nadler et al. [12], was found only in 70% (16/23) of cases, because in 3 patients CD19 and in 4 TdT were not expressed (table 2b).

In the CD10− group the CD24 was present in only 26% (4/15) of leukemias. Furthermore, the CD20 and CyIgM were never demonstrated.

Regarding the myeloid antigens (MyAg) coexpression, the two groups had a different behavior. In the CD10+ leukemias, only five cases (21%) expressed MyAg and only one coexpressed two of them simultaneously (this case was also TdT negative). In the CD 10− cases, 74% demonstrated MyAg and often more than one of them, without any particular difference regarding the CD were frequently found.

In five cases, 3 in the CD10+ and 2 in the CD10− group, an unexpected positivity of CD7 was found. One CD10+ case was TdT−, as well as both CD10− cases.

Table 2a. T ALL immunological findings

Case	Tdt	HLA DR	CD 10	CD 19	CD 24	CD 9	CD 20	Cy IgM	Sm Ig	CD 7
1	+	−	−	−	n	n	n	−	−	+
2	+	−	+	−	−	−	−	−	−	+

Case	CD 5	CD 2	CD 3	CD 11b	CD 13	CD 14	CD 15	CD 33	CDW65 and others
1	n	n	n		−	−	−	−	+
2	+	+	+		−	−	−	−	n

+: > 20 % positive cells; −: < 20 % positive cells; n: not performed

Table 2b. CD 10 positive cases: immunological findings

Case	Tdt	HLA DR	CD 10	CD 19	CD 24	CD 9	CD 20	Cy IgM	Sm Ig	CD 7	CD 5	CD 2	CD 3	CD 11b	CD 13	CD 14	CD 15	CD 33	CDW65 and others
1	+	+	+	n	n	n	n	+	-	n	n	-	n	n	n	n	n	n	n
2	+	+	+	-	+	n	-	-	-	-	-	-	-	n	n	n	n	-	n
3	+	+	+	-	+	-	n	-	-	-	-	n	-	n	n	n	n	-	n
4	n	+	+	+	+	+	-	-	-	-	-	-	-	-	-	-	-	-	n
5	+	+	+	+	+	+	-	+	-	-	-	-	-	n	-	-	-	-	n
6	+	+	+	+	+	+	+	+	-	-	-	-	-	-	-	-	-	-	n
7	n	+	+	-	-	n	-	-	-	+	n	n	n	n	n	n	n	n	-
8	+	+	+	+	+	+	+	+	-	-	-	-	-	-	-	-	-	-	-
9	+	+	+	+	+	+	+	+	-	-	-	-	-	-	-	-	-	-	-
10	+	+	+	+	+	+	+	n	-	n	n	n	n	n	n	n	n	n	+
11	-	+	+	+	+	+	+	-	-	+	-	-	-	-	-	-	-	-	-
12	-	+	+	+	+	+	-	-	-	-	-	-	-	-	-	-	-	-	-
13	-	+	+	n	-	n	-	-	-	-	-	-	-	-	-	-	-	-	-
14	n	+	+	n	+	+	-	+	-	+	-	n	n	n	n	n	n	n	+
15	n	+	+	+	+	+	+	+	-	-	-	-	-	-	-	-	-	-	-
16	+	+	+	+	+	+	+	+	-	-	-	-	-	+	+	+	+	-	-
17	+	+	+	+	+	+	+	n	-	-	n	n	n	n	n	n	n	n	-
18	+	+	+	+	+	+	+	n	-	-	-	-	-	-	-	-	-	-	-
19	+	+	+	+	+	-	+	n	-	-	-	-	-	-	-	-	-	-	-
20	n	+	+	+	n	n	+	n	-	n	n	-	n	n	n	+	n	n	n
21	n	+	+	+	n	n	+	n	-	-	n	-	n	n	n	n	n	+	n
22	n	+	+	+	n	n	+	n	-	-	n	n	n	n	n	n	n	n	n
23	-	+	+	+	+	n	+	n	-	-	-	-	-	-	-	-	-	n	n

+: > 20 % positive cells; –: < 20 % positive cells; n: not performed

Table 2c. CD 10 negative cases: immunological findings

case	Tdt	HLA DR	CD 10	CD 19	CD 24	CD 9	CD 20	Cy IgM	Sm Ig	CD 7	CD 5	CD 2	CD 3	CD 11b	CD 13	CD 14	CD 15	CD 33	CDW 65 and others
1	+	+	–	+	–	+	–	–	–	–	–	–	–	n	+	+	+	–	+
2*	+	+	–	+	–	+	–	–	–	–	–	–	–	–	+	–	+	+	n
3*	+	+	–	+	–	+	–	–	–	–	–	–	–	+	+	–	n	–	+
4	–	+	–	+	–	–	–	–	–	+	–	–	n	–	n	n	–	–	+
5*	+	+	–	+	–	+	–	n	–	n	n	n	n	–	+	+	+	n	–
6	–	+	–	+	n	+	–	n	–	–	n	n	–	–	+	n	+	+	n
7	+	+	–	+	–	+	–	–	–	–	–	–	–	+	+	+	+	+	+
8*	+	+	–	+	n	n	–	n	–	–	–	–	–	n	+	n	n	+	+
9*	+	+	–	+	n	n	–	–	–	–	–	–	–	+	+	+	n	+	n
10	–	+	–	+	–	+	–	–	–	–	–	–	n	–	–	–	–	–	–
11	+	+	–	+	+	+	–	–	–	–	n	–	–	–	–	–	–	–	–
12	–	+	–	–	–	n	–	–	–	–	–	–	n	–	–	n	–	+	–
13*	+	+	–	–	+	–	n	–	–	–	n	–	–	–	–	–	–	–	–
14	+	+	–	+	+	+	n	–	–	+	–	–	–	+	+	+	+	+	+
15	+	+	–	n	n	n	n	–	–	–	–	–	–	+	–	–	+	–	n
16*	+	+	–	+	–	+	n	–	–	–	–	–	–	–	–	–	–	–	–
17	n	+	–	n	–	n	n	n	–	+	–	–	n	–	–	n	–	+	n
18	n	+	–	n	n	n	n	n	–	–	–	–	n	–	n	–	n	n	–
19	n	+	–	+	+	+	n	n	–	–	–	–	n	+	n	–	n	–	n
20	–	+	–	–	–	+	–	–	–	–	–	–	n	–	–	–	+	–	–
21	+	+	–	+	–	+	–	n	–	–	–	–	–	–	n	n	–	+	+
22	–	+	–	n	n	n	n	n	–	–	–	–	n	–	n	–	n	–	n
23	n	+	–	+	n	n	–	–	–	–	–	–	–	–	–	–	n	–	n

+: > 20 % positive cells; –: < 20 % positive cells; n: not performed; *: t(4:11)

Discussion

114 children younger than 1 year of age have entered into the immuno-phenotypic study of AIEOP since 1976. 48 infants were considered eligible for adequate investigation and were evaluated for the present study. The results indicated many differences in immunophenotype between infants and older children. First of all, 15 % of childhood ALL usually show a T cell origin [3, 4, 6], as against 4 % (2 out of 48 infants) in our experience. This has also been registered in previous studies [6, 12], in which rarely T ALL are demonstrated with adequate investigation. All remaining 46 AL were HLA-DR positive, suggesting a B cell origin according to classical classification of ALL. In this group the frequency of Common ALL antigen (CD10) was higher than expected: In fact, in the POG study [6], 14 % of ALL in children younger than 1 year were CD10+ and Ludwig et al. found in the same age group an incidence of 28 % (10/35) [6]. In our study, half of the patients were CALLA+; this high frequency permitted the identification of two homogeneous groups among non-T ALL, CD10+ and CD10-. As it is reported on other casistics, both groups frequently showed positivity to CD19 Ag, usually considered an early marker of B cell differentiation [13]. The CD10+ group, however, presented high frequency of CD24 Ag (96 %). This is in agreement with the incidence reported among CALLA+ leuke-mias both in older children and adults [8]. Surprisingly, albeit previously reported, some CD10+ cases had an unusual phenotype, being CD19 and/or TdT negative. On the other hand, only 26 % of CD10- AL expressed the CD24 Ag; this is a lower incidence than that reported by Ludwig et al. [12].

The unusual positivity to CD7 was found both in the CD10+ and in the CD10- group. In the case of CD10+ A.L., this might be referred to an aberr-ant coexpression of different lineage antigens, while the CD10- cases had an immunological profile that could be consistent also with a non-lymphoid origin, showing TdT negativity, HLA-DR positivity and occasional positiv-ity to other lymphoid markers.

The CD10+ ALL presented a more evoluted phenotype along the B cell lineage, also because of frequent positivity to CD20 and/or CyIgM. On the contrary, these two late B cell markers were absent in all CD10- leuke-mias; this difference confirms the adequacy of our subclassification in iden-tifying two different stages of infant leukemias.

This concept ist reinforced by the finding of myeloid antigens at a dif-ferent frequency between the two groups. The coexpression of lymphoid and myeloid antigen is characteristic of AL in infants [7, 12]. This is one of the criteria proposed for the identification of 'hybrid leukemias' [9], and is also viewed as phenotypic promiscuity on multipotent stem cells [10]. We observed, however, that this coexpression was peculiar of the CD10- group. Among the 20 cases in which myeloid antigens were examined, only 3 cases did not express any of them; on the other hand, 5/19 CD10- AL had MyAg on their surface. On the whole, the antigenic profile mostly observed in our CD10- cases, i.e. TdT+, HLA-DR+, CD19+, CD9+/-, CD24-, CD20-, CyIgM-, weights for an immature population. A similar phenotype was demonstrated in some acute leukemias that showed myeloperoxidase at electron microscopy [1].

We observed that the monoclonal antibody My9 (CD33) was expressed on 7 out of 17 studied cases (41 %); this, however, was not the case among Ludwig's patients [12].

Moreover, 7 of the CD10- cases had the chromosomal translocation t(4:11) and were rearranged for the heavy chain of immunoglobulins. They represent a particular form of 'hybrid' or 'mixed lineage' leukemia, presenting both lymphoid characteristics and monocytoid differentiation capabilities [6, 20]. The prognosis of this cytogenetic abnormality is confirmed in our series and accounts for the unfavourable outcome of the CD10- group. The presence of this translocation, commonly observed in infants, only among the CD10- cases, could further confirm the validity of our distinction. Furthermore, the coexpression of myeloid antigens has been found to be associated with a worse prognosis [18].

In conclusion, the immunological phenotype in infants has only clinical relevance, since it identifies different forms of acute leukemias, in which different therapeutic approaches can be used. The T-ALL and the CD10+ ALL could benefit from anti-lymphoid drugs, while the CD10- group, having the worst outcome, could be treated with aggressive or even experimental therapies (e.g. allogenic bone marrow transplantation, immunotherapy), keeping in mind that anti-myeloid drugs should be the best regimen, because of the possible differentiation into acute myelo-monocytic leukemia.

Summary

Acute leukemia (AL) in infants (less than 12 months of age) is rare and often peculiar in its clinical aspects (high white blood cell count, organomegaly) and biological features (expecially cytogenetics). We analyzed the immunophenotypes of 48 cases that had been adequately examined at various Italian institutions. Only 2 of them were diagnosed as T-ALL. All other cases were HLA-DR+, and about half of them (23 cases) were CD10+. This group had a high frequency of CD19, CD24 and TdT positivity, thus confirming the pertinence to B-cell lineage. They were also often CD20+ and/or CyIgM+ (B mature phenotype). The 23 CD10-negative cases were also frequently TdT+ and CD19+, but were mostly CD24-, CD20-, CyIgM-. The coexpression of myeloid antigens on CD10- leukemias reinforces the possible origin from a more primitive cell and justifies the definition of 'hybrid' AL. Moreover, particular 'hybrid' chromosomal translocations, such as t(4;11), were found in 7 of the CD10-negative cases.

Acknowledgement

The authors wish to thank Mrs. F.Bonan, M.G. Giacometti, C.Molena for technical assistance.

References

1 Basso G, Putti MC, Catoretti G, Consolini R, Galdiolo D, Guglielmi C, Messina C, Milanesi C, Testi AM, Zillo Monte Xillo M, Zulian F, Foá R: Heterogeneity of TdT+, HLA-DR+ acute leukemia: immunological, immunocytochemical and clinical evidence of lymphoid and myeloid origin. Eur J Hematol 1987;38:111–116.

2 Bennet JM, Catovsky D, Daniel MT, Flandrin G, Galton DAG, Gralnick HR, Sultan C: Proposal for the classification of the acute leukemias. Br J Haematol 1976;33:451–458.

3 Brouet JC, Valensi F, Daniel MT, Flandrin G, Prud'Homme JL, Seligmann M: Immunological classification of acute lymphoblastic leukemias: evaluation of its clinical significance in a hundred patients. Br J Haematol, 1976;33:319–328.

4 Chessels JM, Hardistry RM, Rapson MT, Greaves MF: Acute lymphoblastic leukemia in children: classification and prognosis. Lancet 1977;II:1307–1309.

5 Crist W, Cleary ML, Grossi CE: Acute leukemia associated with the t(4;11) chromosomal rearrangement exhibits B lineage and monocytic characteristics. Blood; 1985;66:33–38.

6 Crist W, Pullen J, Boyett J, Falletta J, Van Eys J, Borowitz M, Jackson J, Dowell B, Frankel L, Quddus F, Ragab A, Vietti T: Clinical and biological features predict a poor prognosis in acute lymphoid leukemias in infants: A pediatric oncology group study. Blood 1986;67:135–140.

7 Dinndorf PA, Reaman GH: Acute lymphoblastic leukemia in infants: evidence for B cell origin of disease by use of monoclonal antibody phenotyping. Blood 1986;68:975–978.

8 Foá R, Migone N, Fierro MT, Basso G, Lusso P, Putti MC, Giubellino MC, Saitta M, Miniero R, Casorati G, Gavosto F: Genotypic characterization of common acute lymphoblastic leukemia may improve the phenotypic classification. Exp Hematol 1987;15:942–945.

9   Gale RP, Ben-Bassat I: Hybrid acute leukemia. Br J Haematol 1987;65:261–264.
10 Greaves MF, Chan LC, Furley AJW, Watt SM, Molgaard HV: Lineage promiscuity in hemopoetic differentiation and leukemia. Blood 1986;67:1–11.
11 Ludwig WD, Bartram CR, Ritter J, Raghavachar A, Hiddemann W, Heil G, Harbott J, Seibt-Jung H, Teichmann IV, Riehm H: Ambiguous phenotypes and genotypes in 16 children with acute leukemia as characterized by multiparameter analysis. Blood 1988;71:1518–1528.
12 Ludwig WD, Bartram CR, Harbott J, Koeller U, Haas OA, Hansen-Hagge T, Heil G, Seibt-Jung H, Teichmann JV, Ritter J, Knapp W, Gadner H, Thiel E, Riehm H: Phenotypic and genotypic heterogeneity in infant acute leukemia I. Acute lymphoblastic leukemia. Leuk 1989;6:431–439.
13 Nadler LM, Korsmayer S, Anderson KC: B cell origin of non-T acute lymphoblastic leukemia. A model for discrete stages of neoplastic and normal pre-B cell differentiation. J Clin Invest 1984;74:332–340.
14 Paolucci G, Masera G, Vecchi V, Marsoni S, Pession A, Zurlo MG (AIEOP): Treating childhood acute lymphoblastic leukemia: summary of ten years experience in Italy. Med Ped Oncol, 1989;17:83–91.
15 Pui CH, Raimondi SC, Murphy SB, Ribeiro RC, Kalwinsky DK, Dahl GV, Crist WM, Williams DL: An analysis of leukemic cell chromosomal features in infants. Blood, 1989;69:1289–1293.
16 Reaman G, Zelter P, Bleyer WA, Amendola B, Level C, Hammond D: Acute lymphoblastic leukemia in infants less than one year of age: a cumulative experience of the Children Cancer Study Group. J Clin Oncol 1985;3:1513.
17 Scroggs M, Boyett J, Pullen DJ, Jackson J, Russel E, Crist W, Borowitz M: Clinicopathologic significance of immunophenotypic subgroups of B lineage acute lymphocytic leukemia (ALL). A pediatric oncology group (POG) study. Proc Am Ass Cancer Res 1986;27:201.
18 Sobol RE, Mick R, Royston I, Davey FR, Ellison RR, Newman R, Cuttner J, Griffin JD, Collins H, Nelson DA, Bloomfield CD: Clinical importance of myeloid antigen expression in adult acute lymphoblastic leukemia. N Engl J Med 1987;316:1111–1117.
19 Stark B, Vogel R, Cohen IJ, Umiel T, Mammon Z, Rechavi G, Kaplinsky C, Potaznik D, Dvir A, Yaniv Y, Goshen Y, Katzir N, Ramot B, Zaizov R: Biologic and cytogenetic characteristics of leukemias in infants. Cancer 1989;63:117–125.
20 Strong CR, Korsmeyer SJ, Parkin JL, Arthur DC, Kersey JH: Human acute leukemia cell line with the t(4;11) chromosomal rearrangement exhibits B cell lineage and monocytic characteristics. Blood 1985;65:21–31.

Dr. Giuseppe Basso, Dipartimento di Pediatria dell'Università di Padova,
Via Giustiniani, 3, I-35128 Padova (Italy)

Contrib Oncol. Basel, Karger, 1990, vol 41, pp 46–49.

Phenotypic and Genotypic Heterogeneity in Infant Acute Leukemia[1] (Abstract)

W. D. Ludwig[a], *U. Köller*[b], *C. R. Bartram*[c], *J. Harbott*[d], *O. A. Haas*[e], *J. Ritter*[f], *U. Creutzig*[f], *H. Gadner*[e], *H. Riehm*[g]

[a] Department of Hematology/Oncology, Klinikum Steglitz, Berlin
[b] Institute of Immunology, University of Vienna, Austria
[c] Section of Molecular Biology, Department of Pedatrics II, University of Ulm, FRG
[d] Department of Pediatrics, University of Gießen, FRG
[e] Children's Cancer Research Institute, St. Anna Children's Hospital, Vienna, Austria
[f] Department of Pediatrics, University of Münster, FRG
[g] Department of Pediatrics, Hannover Medical School, FRG

Clinical and biological features of acute leukemia in infants differ markedly from those in older children and are probably associated in part with the poor prognosis described for these patients.

In order to enhance our knowledge on the etiology of the disease and to provide a biologic explanation for its worse treatment outcome, we studied the blast cells from a large series of infants aged < 1 year with acute unclassifiable leukemia (n=1), acute lymphoblastic leukemia (ALL) (n=44), acute myeloid leukemia (AML) (n=26), and acute leukemia with coexistence of two separate cell populations, one with lymphoid and the other with myeloid features (n=3). Leukemic blasts from these patients were analyzed at the time of initial diagnosis with an extensive panel of monoclonal antibodies recognizing myeloid and lymphoid-associated antigens, and immunophenotypic features were correlated with genotypic findings.

A CD10 (common ALL antigen)-negative, CD19-positive pre-pre-B ALL phenotype was observed in 28 of 44 infants with ALL. Twenty-two of

---

[1] This work was partly supported by the DAL/GPO, the Deutsche Forschungsgemeinschaft, the Deutsche Krebshilfe, and the 'Fonds zur Förderung der wissenschaftlichen Forschung in Österreich'

them had blast cells coexpressing myeloid-associated markers such as CD15 and/or CDw65. Seven patients showed a typical common ALL, six a pre-B ALL, one a B-ALL, and one a pre-T ALL phenotype (table 1).

Immunoglobulin (Ig) and T-cell receptor (TCR) β-, γ-, and δ-chain gene analysis of 39 infants with ALL revealed Ig heavy-chain gene rearrangements in all but one patient with B-cell precursor (BCP) ALL; there was evidence of clonal evolution in six of the infants and K-light-chain gene rearrangement in 6 of them. One patient with a pre-T ALL phenotype disclosed clonal TCR β-, γ-, and δ-chain gene rearrangements. 'Inappropriate' TCR gene rearrangements (TCR δ > TCR γ > TCR β) were detected in 22 infants with BCP ALL (table 2). Structural abnormalities affecting the long arm of chromosome 11 at band q23, most frequently due to the t(4;11), were observed in 10 infants with a CD10-negative pre-pre-B ALL phenotype and frequent overlapping of CD15 and/or CDw65 antigen expression.

Bone-marrow examination at diagnosis showed lymphoblasts with a CD10-negative pre-pre-B ALL phenotype in 2 patients and coexpression of myeloid antigens in one of them. Shortly after initiation of induction chemotherapy for ALL, large blasts with monocytoid features appeared in the peripheral blood of both patients, and immunophenotyping confirmed their monocytic origin. Molecular analysis revealed Ig heavy-chain gene rearrangement in the one patient and germline configuration of all Ig and

Table 1. Immunophenotypic features in 44 infants with ALL

Immunophenotype	No. of patients
Acute 'unclassifiable' leukemia (AUL)	1
HLA-DR$^+$; pan-B, pan-T and myeloid AG$^-$	
Pre-pre-B ALL (null ALL)	6
TdT$^+$, HLA-DR$^+$, CD19$^+$, CD10$^-$, myeloid AG$^-$	
Myeloid AG$^+$ pre-pre-B ALL (My$^+$ pre-pre-B ALL)	22*
TdT$^+$, HLA-DR$^+$, CD19$^+$, CD10$^-$, CDw65$^{+/-}$, CD15$^{+/-}$, CD13/33$^-$	
Common ALL	7
TdT$^+$, HLA-DR$^+$, CD19$^+$, CD10$^+$, myeloid AG$^-$	
Pre-B ALL	6
TdT$^+$, HLA-DR$^+$, CD19$^+$, CD10$^+$, cyIgM$^+$, myeloid AG$^-$	
B-ALL	1
TdT$^+$, HLA-DR$^+$, CD19$^+$, CD20$^+$, sIg$^+$, CD10$^+$, myeloid AG$^-$	
Pre-T ALL	1
TdT$^+$, HLA-DR$^-$, CD10$^+$, CD7$^+$, CD5$^+$, CD2$^-$, myeloid AG$^-$	

* Myeloperoxidase negative at the ultrastructural level in 5/5 patients.

TCR genes in the other one. Cytogenetic investigations disclosed t(11;19) and t(1;11) respectively. The majority of blast cells from a third patient with distinct blast populations displayed myeloid cell surface antigens (CD33, CDw65), whereas a minority (about 30 %) of morphologically lymphoblastic cells showed a typical common ALL phenotype. No rearrangements of Ig and TCR genes were detected in this infant, and cytogenetic findings were not available.

Immunophenotyping revealed myelomonocytic features in 19 of 26 infants with AML. Monoblastic leukemia was diagnosed in 12 of these 19 patients, and blast cells expressed nearly all myeloid antigens tested, including CD15. Clear-cut expression of CD14 antigen was observed in 9 of 12 infants with monoblastic features. Erythroleukemia with a rather mature phenotype, as indicated by a high proportion of glycophorin-A-positive cells, was identified in 2 patients and acute megakaryocytic leukemia with a high number of glycoprotein-IIb/IIIa (CD41) – or IIIa-positive blasts in 5 patients (table 3). Ig and TCR gene analyses performed in 20 of 26 infants with AML disclosed rearrangement of Ig heavy chain sequences in 5 cases, one exhibiting multiple rearranged fragments. Three of these patients showed additional TCR δ-chain gene rearrangements, while Ig K-light-chain, TCR β- as well as TCR γ-chain were in germline position in all cases analyzed. Chromosomal analysis was successfully performed in 20 patients, and, as in infant ALL, chromosome 11 was by far the mostly affected chromosome. It was involved in 10 of 18 abnormal cases and was significantly associated with monoblastic features.

Table 2. Immunophenotypic and genotypic features in infants with ALL

Immunophenotype	No. of patients	Gene rearrangement				
		IgH	IgL (K)	Tβ	Tγ	Tδ
AUL	1	1/1[*]	0/1	0/1	1/1	0/1
Pre-pre-B ALL	6	5/5[**]	0/5	1/5	0/5	2/5
My[+] pre-pre-B ALL	22	22/22[+]	3/22	3/22	3/22	8/21
Common ALL	7	4/4[++]	1/4	1/4	2/4	4/4
Pre-B ALL	6	5/6	2/6	3/6	1/5	5/6
Pre-T ALL	1	0/1	0/1	1/1	1/1	1/1

[*] Rearranged genes/patients examined.
[**] Multiple rearranged fragments in 2 patients.
[+] Multiple rearranged fragments in 3 patients.
[++] Multiple rearranged fragments in 1 patient.

Table 3. Immunophenotypic features in 26 infants with AML

Immunophenotype	No. of patients
AML	7
HLA-DR$^+$, CDw65$^+$, CD13$^{+/-}$, CD33$^{+/-}$, CD14$^-$, TdT$^{-/+}$	
AMOL	12
HLA-DR$^+$, CDw65$^+$, CD13$^{+/-}$, CD33$^{+/-}$, CD14$^{+/-}$, TdT$^-$	
Acute erythroleukemia	2
CD13$^{+/-}$, CD33$^{+/-}$, glycophorin A$^+$	
Acute megakaryocytic leukemia	5
CD13$^{+/-}$, CD33$^{+/-}$, CD41$^+$, TdT$^{-/+}$	

In conclusion, our data indicate that infant acute leukemias are heterogeneous with respect to immunophenotypic and genotypic features and confirm other recent reports in demonstrating a high incidence of very early BCP ALL and acute monoblastic leukemia. The frequently encountered biologic characteristics – including coexpression of myeloid antigens within the most immature BCP ALL subgroup, coexistence of lymphoid and myeloid blast cell populations and rearrangements involving q23 region of chromosome 11-probably reflect the immature developmental stage of blast cells in most infant acute leukemias, which may contribute to the poor treatment outcome of these patients.

PD Dr. Wolf-Dieter Ludwig, Abteilung für Innere Medizin,
Universitätsklinikum Steglitz, Hindenburgdamm 30, D-1000 Berlin 45

Contrib Oncol. Basel, Karger, 1990, vol 41, pp 50–56.

Cytogenetic Findings in Acute Leukemias of Infants[1]

J. Harbott[a], *J. Ritterbach*[a], *U. Creutzig*[b], *H. Riehm*[c], *F. Lampert*[a]

[a] Oncocytogenetic Laboratory, Children's Hospital, University of Gießen
[b] Children's Hospital, University of Münster
[c] Department of Pediatrics, Hannover Medical School, FRG

Zusammenfassung

Sowohl die klinischen als auch die zellbiologischen Merkmale von Säuglingen mit akuter Leukämie unterscheiden sich erheblich von denen älterer Kinder. Die zytogenetischen Befunde aus Knochenmarkszellen von 28 Säuglingen mit ALL und 16 mit ANLL machen deutlich, daß Aberrationen des langen Arms von Chromosom 11 in der Bande q23 die häufigsten Veränderungen (ca. 60 %) in akuten Säuglingsleukämien darstellen. Andere strukturelle oder numerische Aberrationen traten dagegen selten auf. Der Vergleich dieser Ergebnisse mit denen von Kindern, die älter als ein Jahr sind, zeigt signifikante Unterschiede. Die Pathogenese der Säuglingsleukämie könnte durch ein Chromosomenrearrangement in einer pluripotenten Vorläuferzelle zustande kommen, die sowohl lymphatische als auch myeloische Differenzierungsmöglichkeiten hat.

Introduction

Large retrospective reviews dealing with acute leukemia in infants have noted the adverse clinical features of children younger than one year [1, 2]. These features are higher WBC, an increased incidence of hepatosplenomegaly, and central nervous disease at diagnosis, and may be associated with the poor treatment response in these children.

Also, the biological features in infants such as immunophenotype, molecular rearrangements and cytogenetic abnormalities differ from those found in older children [2–9].

Despite the knowledge of the unique features in infant leukemia, there are only a few reports of cytogenetic data of infants [7, 10, 11]. Cytogenetic

---

[1] Dedicated to Professor Dr. P. Koch, Marburg, on the occasion of his 60th birthday

results may not only give more information about pathogenesis, but may also be a diagnostic tool in infant leukemia. We therefore wish to report the leukemo-cytogenetic data of 44 children younger than one year of age.

Materials and Methods

Bone marrow samples, mostly received by mail (80–90 %), were washed twice in RPMI 1640 and then either prepared directly and/or incubated in RPMI 1640 + 20 % FCS for a 24-h culture. The cell suspension was then brought to hypotonic solution (KC1, 15 min) and fixed in methanol-acetic acid (3:1). After being washed six to eight times, the cells were dropped on a cold wet slide to spread the metaphases. G-banding was done after a trypsin pretreatment (10–15 sec) 3–5 days later.

From January 1984 to April 1989 we received 1074 bone marrow samples of children with newly diagnosed ALL (n = 866) and ANLL (n = 208) for cytogenetic investigations. All patients were treated according to one of the West-German multicenter therapy studies BFM-ALL, BFM-AML, and CoALL, respectively. 627 (59 %) of the mailed specimens could be analysed successfully, 481 (56 %) of patients with ALL and 146 (70 %) with ANLL. Among these patients 44 (7.0 %) were infants, 28 (5.8 %) with ALL and 16 (11.0 %) with ANLL.

Results

In contrast to the patients who were older than one year, infants showed a higher incidence of abnormal karyotypes in their leukemic cells (tables 1, 2). Whereas 22/28 (78.6 %) of the infants with ALL had structural and/or numerical aberrations, the percentage was even higher in infants with ANLL (13/16; 81.2 %). In contrast to that, the incidence of abnormal

Table 1. Karyotype aberrations in ALL in infants and older children

Ploidy	Infants		> 1 year		Total	
	abs	%	abs	%	abs	%
Hypodiploid	0	0	16	3.5	16	3.3
Diploid	6	21.4	195	43.0	201	41.8
Pseudodiploid	18	64.3	98	21.6	116	24.1
Hyperdiploid 47–50	3	10.7	44	9.7	47	9.8
Hyperdiploid > 50	1	3.6	100	22.1	101	21.0
Total	28	5.8	453	94.2	481	

karyotypes was much lower in older children with ALL (57.0 %) and ANLL (70.8 %), respectively. Whereas the difference was significant in ALL (p<0.0001), it was not in ANLL (p = 0.7148), because of the small number of patients. Especially infants with pseudodiploid karyotypes were more frequent in both groups.

Comparing the appearance of non-random and random chromosomal rearrangements, the band 11q23 was most frequently found to be involved in aberrations of infant leukemias (tables 3, 4). 13/22 (59.1 %) of the infants with ALL and 7/12 (58.3 %) with ANLL showed this kind of abnormality. The t(4;11) (q21;q23) appeared in 11 infants (50.0 %) with ALL, the t(9;11)

Table 2. Karyotype aberrations in ANLL in infants and older children

Ploidy	Infants		>1 year		Total	
	abs	%	abs	%	abs	%
Hypodiploid	1	6.2	4	3.1	5	3.4
Diploid	3	18.8	38	29.2	41	28.1
Pseudodiploid	8	50.0	52	40.0	60	41.1
Hyperdiploid	4	25.0	36	27.7	40	27.4
Total	16	11.0	130	89.0	146	

Table 3. Non-random chromosomal aberrations in ALL of infants and older children

Aberration	Infants		>1 year		Total	
	abs	%	abs	%	abs	%
t (1;19)	0	0	9	3.9	9	3.6
t (8;14)	1	4.5	11	4.8	12	5.2
t (9;22)	0	0	9	3.9	9	3.6
der (14q11)	1	4.5	9	3.9	10	4.0
del (6q)	1	4.5	8	3.5	9	3.6
del (9p)	0	0	8	3.5	8	3.2
del (12p)	0	0	4	1.7	4	1.9
>50 chr.	1	4.5	107	46.3	108	42.7
Random aberr.	5	22.7	59	25.5	64	25.3
t (4;11)	11	50.0	4	1.7	15	5.9
der (11q23)	2	9.1	3	1.3	5	2.0
Total	22		231		253	

(p22;q23) in 1 infant (8.3 %) with ANLL, whereas 2 infants with ALL (9.1 %) and 6 with ANLL (50.0 %) showed other abnormalities involving the band q23 of chromosome 11, such as deletions or translocations with different chromosomes. 11q23-aberrations in children older than one year were very rare (3.0 % in ALL and 20.9 % in ANLL), and the frequency differed significantly from that of infancy (ALL: $p < 0.0001$; ANLL: $p = 0.008$).

Discussion

Chromosomal aberrations involving the band 11q23 are the most frequent abnormalities in leukemic blast cells of infants either in ALL or ANLL in this study. The frequency of these rearrangements is about 6.5 times higher than in older children. These findings are confirmed by Pui et al. [7], who described 11q23-aberrations in half of the investigated infants, and also Abe et al. [10], Abe and Sandberg [12] and Raimondi et al. [13] noted a higher frequency in infants. Among the 18 patients younger than one year, however, cytogenetically investigated by Stark et al. [11], only two had rearrangements of 11q23.

Table 4. Non-random chromosomal aberrations in ANLL of infants and older children

Aberration	Infants		> 1 year		Total	
	abs	%	abs	%	abs	%
t (8;21)	0	0.0	16	17.6	16	15.5
t (15;17)	0	0.0	6	6.6	6	5.8
inv (16)	0	0.0	6	6.6	6	5.8
t (9;22)	0	0.0	0	0.0	0	0.0
del (9q)	0	0.0	1	1.1	1	1.0
del (20q)	0	0.0	0	0.0	0	0.0
−5/del (5q)	1	8.3	2	2.2	3	2.9
−7/del (7q)	1	8.3	1	1.1	2	1.9
+8	1	8.3	13	14.3	14	13.6
+4	0	0.0	1	1.1	1	1.0
Random aberr.	2	16.7	26	28.6	28	27.2
t(9;11)	1	8.3	11	12.1	12	11.7
der (11q23)	6	50.0	8	8.8	14	13.6
Total	12	100.0	91	100.0	103	100.0

The findings of this study concerning the type of 11q23-aberrations conform widely with Pui's results [7]. The t(9;11), however, which is typical for ANLL-M5, was more often found in children older than one year, even if the percentage was only slightly higher (8.3 % in infants versus 12.1 % in older children). This fact might be due to the small number of patients with ANLL.

The adverse clinical markers of infant leukemia such as splenomegaly, high WBC, and CNS disease may be one reason for the poor outcome of these children. On the other hand, the frequency of pseudodiploidy is about 4 times higher in infants than in older children. The appearance of structural aberrations, especially translocations, was previously shown to be a poor prognostic factor [14–16]. Hyperdiploidy with more than 50 chromosomes, however, a well-known indicator for good prognosis, was only found in one infant in this series, and was never described by other authors [7,10,11]. Lack of hyperdiploidy and the high frequency of pseudodiploidy may be the biological reasons of the poor outcome of infant acute leukemia.

Most of the non-random rearrangements of 11q23 are described in both types of acute leukemia. Pui et al. [7] found patients with t(9;11) mostly in ANLL, but also in ALL. From our laboratory, patients with t(4;11) associated with ppB-ALL, mixed leukemia, and even ANLL-M5 (17) and t(11;19) associated with mixed leukemia [18] were reported. This great variety of the immunophenotype was assumed to be caused by a chromosomal rearrangement in a multipotent progenitor cell with potential for both myeloid and lymphoid differentiation [19–22].

The translocation of the oncogene c-ets-1 [23], which is located in 11q23 [24], was thought to cause leukemogenesis. Rearrangements of this gene, however, have not been found in infant blast cells [4], and further studies have to find out the role of 11q23-aberrations in infants.

Summary

Clinical as well as biological features of infants differ widely from those of children older than one year. Cytogenetic analysis of bone marrow cells of 28 infants with ALL and 16 with ANLL made obvious that rearrangements involving the long arm of chromosome 11 band q23 were the most frequent abnormalities (about 60 %) in acute leukemia of infants. Other structural or numerical aberrations appeared only rarely. The comparison of these results with those of older children showed significant differences. The pathogenesis of infant leukemia may be caused by chromosomal rearrangements in pluripotent progenitor cells with potential for both myeloid and lymphoid differentiation.

Acknowledgement

This study was supported by the Kind-Philipp-Stiftung and the Parents' Initiative Gießen.

References

1   Reaman G, Zeltzer P, Bleyer WA, Amendola B, Level C, Sather H, Hammond D: Acute lymphoblastic leukemia in infants less than one year of age: a cumulative experience of the children's cancer study group. J Clin Oncol 1985;3:1513–1521.

2   Crist W, Pullen J, Boyett J, Falletta J, van Eys J, Borowitz M, Jackson J, Dowell B, Frankel L, Quddus F, Ragab A, Vietti T: Clinical and biological features predict a poor prognosis in acute lymphoid leukemias in infants: a pediatric oncology group study. Blood 1986;67:135–140.

3   Dinndorf PA, Reaman GH: Acute lymphoblastic leukemia in infants: evidence for cell origin of disease by use of monoclonal antibody phenotyping. Blood 1986;68:975–978.

4   Katz F, Malcolm S, Gibbons B, Tilly R, Lam G, Robertson ME, Czepulkowski B, Chessels J: Cellular and molecular studies on infant null acute lymphoblastic leukemia. Blood 1988;71:1438–1447.

5   Nagasaka M, Maeda S, Maeda H, Chen HL, Kita K, Mabuchi O, Misu H, Matsuo T, Sugiyama T: Four cases of t(4;11) acute leukemia and its myelomonocytic nature in infants. Blood 1983;61:1174–1181.

6   Kaneko Y, Maseki N, Takasaki N, Sakurai M, Hyashi Y, Nakazawa S, Mori T, Sakurai M, Takeda T, Shikano T, Hiyoshi Y: Clinical and hematologic characteristics in acute leukemia with 11q23 translocations. Blood 1986;67:484–491.

7   Pui CH, Raimondi SC, Murphy SB, Ribeiro RC, Kalwinsky DK, Dahl GV, Crist WM, Williams DL: An analysis of leukemic cell chromosomal features in infants. Blood 1987;69:1289–1293.

8   Felix CA, Reaman GH, Korsmeyer SJ, Hollis GF, Dinndorf PA, Wright JJ, Kirsch IR: Immunoglobin and T cell receptor gene configuration in acute lymphoblastic leukemia in infancy. Blood 1987;70:536–541.

9   Rechavi G, Brok-Simoni F, Katzir N, Mandel M, Umiel T, Stark B, Zaizov R, Ben-Bassat I, Ramot B: More than two immunoglobulin heavy chain J regions genes in the majority of infant leukemia. Leuk 1988;2:347–350.

10 Abe R, Ryan D, Cecalupo A, Cohen H, Sandberg AA: Cytogenetic findings in congenital leukemia: Case report and review of the literature. Cancer Genet Cytogenet 1983;9:139–144.

11 Stark B, Vogel R, Cohen IJ, Umiel T, Mommon Z, Rechavi G, Kaplinsky C, Potaznik D, Dvir A, Yaniv Y, Goshen Y, Katzir N, Ramot B, Zaizov R: Biologic and cytogenetic characteristics of leukemia in infants. Cancer 1989;63:117–125.

12 Abe R, Sandberg AA: (1984) Significance of abnormalities involving chromosomal segment 11q23–25 in acute leukemia. Cancer Genet Cytogenet 1984;13:121–127.

13 Raimondi SC, Peiper SC, Kitchingman GR, Behm FG, Williams DL, Hancock ML, Mirro J: Childhood acute lymphoblastic leukemia with chromosomal breakpoints 11q23. Blood 1989;73:1627–1634.

14   The Third International Workshop on Chromosomes in Leukemia: Cancer Genet Cytogenet 1980;4:96–110.

15   Williams DL, Harber J, Murphy SB, Lok AT, Kalwinsky DK, Rivera G, Melvin SL, Stass S, Dahl GV: Chromosomal translocations play a unique role in influencing prognosis in childhood acute lymphoblastic leukemia. Blood 1986;68:205–212.

16   Harbott J, Ritterbach J, Janka-Schaub G, Ludwig WD, Reiter A, Riehm H, Lampert F: Cytogenetics of childhood acute lymphoblastic leukemia in multicenter trials. Haematol Blood Transfus 1990;33:451–458.

17   Lampert F, Harbott J, Ludwig WD, Bartram CR, Ritter J, Gerein V, Neidhardt M, Mertens R, Graf N, Riehm H: Acute leukemia with chromosome translocation (4;11): 7 new patients and analysis of 71 cases. Blut 1987;54:325–335.

18   Fengler R, Baumgarten E, Buchmann S, Creutzig U, Harbott J, Ludwig WD, Henze G: Biklonale Leukämie (0-ALL/AMol) mit 11;19 Translokation und Trisomie X bei einem 8 Monate alten Mädchen. Klin Pädiat 1986;198:178–182.

19   Mirro J, Kitchingman G, Williams DL, Lauzo GJ, Lin CC, Calihan T, Zipf TF: Clincal and laboratory characteristics of acute leukemia with the 4;11 translocation. Blood 1986;67:689–697.

20   Ludwig WD, Bartram CR, Ritter J, Raghavachar A, Hiddemann W, Heil G, Harbott J, Seibt-Jung H, Teichmann JV, Riehm H: Ambigous phenotypes and genotypes in 16 children with acute leukemia as characterized by multiparameter analysis. Blood 1988;71:1518–1528.

21   Secker-Walker LM, Stewart EL, Chan L, O'Callaghan U, Chessells J: The (4;11) translocation in acute leukaemia of childhood: The importance of additional chromosomal aberrations. Br J Haematol 1985;61:101–111.

22   De Braekeleer M: t(4;11) translocation-assocciated acute leukemia: An update. Cancer Genet Cytogenet 1986;23:333–335.

23   Sacchi N, Watson DK, Guerts van Kessel HM, Hagemeijer A, Kersey J, Drabkin HD, Patterson D, Papas TS: HU-ets-1 and Hu-ets-2 genes are transposed in acute leukemia with (4;11) and (8;21) translocations. Science 1986;231:379–382.

24   DeTaisne C, Gegonne A, Stehelin D: Chromosomal localization of the human proto-oncogene c-ets. Nature 1984;310:581–583.

Dr. Jochen Harbott, Universitäts-Kinderpoliklinik,
Feulgenstraße 12, D-6300 Gießen (FRG)

Contrib Oncol. Basel, Karger, 1990, vol 41, pp 57–64.

T-cell Receptor Delta Gene Configuration
in Acute Lymphoblastic Leukemia of Infancy

A. Biondi [a], *V. Rossi* [a], *S. Benvestito* [a], *P. Francia di Celle* [b], *G. Basso* [c], *N. Migone* [d], *R. Foa* [b]

[a] Department of Pediatrics, University of Milano, E.O.G., Monza
[b] Department of Biomedical Science and Human Oncology, University of Turin
[c] Department of Pediatrics, University of Padua
[d] Department of Genetics, Biology and Clinical Medicine, University of Turin, Italy

Zusammenfassung

Bei 21 Säuglingen mit ALL wurden in den Leukämiezellen die Immunglobulin(Ig)-Schwerketten, Kappa-Leichtketten und die T-Zellrezeptor (TCR) Beta-, Gamma- und Delta-Gene untersucht. Alle 21 Fälle wiesen Leukämiezelloberflächenantigene des B-Zell Vorläufer-Phänotyps auf. Mit einer Ausnahme fanden sich in allen Fällen Rearrangements der Ig-Schwerkettengene. Die Analyse der Ig-Genkonfiguration zeigte bei 5 von 21 Fällen (23 %) vielfach rearrangierte Fragmente variabler autoradiographischer Intensitäten. Bei 3 Säuglingen wurden rearrangierte Ig-Kappa-Leichtkettensequenzen beobachtet. Rearrangements von TCR-Gamma und TCR-Beta traten nur bei 2 Patienten auf, unterschiedlich zu den sonst bei B-Zell Vorläufer ALL im Kindesalter erhobenen Befunden. Neue Banden, TCR Delta entsprechend, fanden sich bei 7 von 20 analysierten Fällen (35 %). Zwei Arten von TCR Delta Rearrangement, ein VDD- und ein DD-Typ, konnten beobachtet werden, und beide scheinen von einem «Partial joining» herzurühren. Diese TCR-Delta-Analysen unterstreichen die Vermutung, daß die ALL im Säuglingsalter allgemein von einer früheren Entwicklungsstufe des Lymphzellsystems entspringt im Vergleich zur ALL im höheren Kindesalter.

Introduction

Despite the considerable improvement in the outcome of childhood acute lymphoblastic leukemia (ALL), the leukemia of infancy is still associated with a poor treatment response [1, 2]. Several biological features of infant ALL have been analyzed and compared with those of older children ALL, in order to gain some biological explanation for its poor prognosis. The results of these studies suggest that ALL of infancy originate mostly in the very early stage of B-cell progenitors which do not express CD10 and are usually characterized by chromosomal rearrangements of band 11q23 [3–7]. Based on the analysis of Immunoglobulin and T-Cell receptor (TCR) genes, it has been suggested that at the molecular genetic level, ALL in infancy represents an earlier stage of lymphocyte development than observed in B cell precursor ALL of children [6].

A new TCR chain gene, TCR delta, has been recently described [8]. It appears to rearrange earlier than beta and alpha during T-cell development, paralleling or possibly preceding the rearrangement and expression of the gamma locus [9]. Taking advantage of the availability of V and J probes for the delta locus, we have examined a series of infant ALL for the DNA configuration at this region, and compared it with with the arrangement of the gamma and beta loci.

Results and Discussion

The 21 patients analyzed ranged in age from 5 days to 12 months. 55 % of the infants presented white blood counts (WBC) $>100 \times 10^9/l$. The majority (56 %) disclosed a CD10 negative pre-pre-B phenotype, with expression of CD19, a variable expression of CD24, and mostly Tdt positive. Cytogenetic data were available in 11 of the 21 patients (52 %). Karyotype abnormalities were detected in 6 cases (54 %). The translocation t(4;11) (q21;937) was found in 3 out of 6 cases.

The main results of genotypic analysis of the 21 patients are summarized in table 1. 20 of 21 patients showed a rearrangement of at least one allele of the Ig heavy chain gene. Multiple rearranged fragments of variable autoradiographic intensities were observed in patients 1, 3, 9, 10 and 14. This observation indicates the presence of different leukemic subclones that evolved from a common leukemic stem cell. This hypothesis is sustained by cytogenetic investigations, showing a single chromosomal aberration, t(4;11), in patient 10, and the presence of a monoclonal TCR delta gene rearrangement common for all leukemic cells analyzed in cases 3 and 14. In patients 10 and 14 we observed rearranged Ig k light chain sequences. The overall incidence (23 %) of multiple rearranged fragments for Ig heavy-chain genes in the caselist analyzed is similar to the one recently observed by Ludwig et al. [10]. The correlation between the presence of more than two u heavy-chain genes and a poor response to treatment, as recently reported [7], will require a larger number of patients and a longer follow-up in order to be confirmed.

Following BamHI and EcoRI analysis, rearrangements of TCR beta and TCR gamma were found in 2 of the 21 patients analyzed. The configuration of the TCR gamma chain gene was determined by probing BamHI and EcoRI-cut DNA with the J gamma-1 probe which recognizes both J gamma-1 and J gamma-2 segments. The gamma chain was rearranged in one case with the use of the C gamma-1 and V gamma-9 gene segments (data not shown). The concomitant rearrangement at the TCR loci has been commonly reported in B-cell precursor ALL (both common and 'null' ALL) [11]. In a recent analysis of 75 children with B-cell precursor ALL, we found that TCR gamma and beta chain genes were rearranged in 46 % and 28 % of the cases evaluated [12]. The lower incidence of TCR gamma and beta gene involvement observed in infant ALL indicates a significant difference at molecular genetic level between the disease in the infants and in children, confirming previous finding by Felix et al. [6].

Table 1. Immunoglobulin and T cell receptor gene configuration in infant ALL

Patient No.	IG heavy	IG light	T cell receptor gene		
	JH	K	$T\beta$	$T\gamma$	$T\delta$
1	R/R/R	G	G	G	G
2	R/D	G	G	G	G/R
3	R/R/R	G/R	G	G	G/R
4	R/R	G	G	G	G
5	R/D	G/R	G	G	G
6	R/R	G	G	G	G
7	R/D	G	G	G/R	G/R
8	G	G	G	G	G
9	R/R/R	G	G	G	G
10	R/R/R	G/R	G	G	G
11	R/R/g	G	G	G	G/R
12	R/D	G	G	G	G
13	G/R	G	G	G	G
14	R/R/R	G	G	G	G/R
15	R/R	G	G	G	N.D
16	R/R	G	G	G	G/R
17	R/R/g	G	G/R	G	G/R
18	G/R	N.D.	G	G	G
19	G/R	N.D.	G	G	G/D
20	R/D	G	G	G	G
21	R/R/g	G	G	G	G

G: germline configuration; D: deleted; N.D: not done

Figure 1 shows a schematic restriction map of the delta locus. We used different probes to determine the structure of the delta locus: The cTH2 probe that contains the C delta region splice to J delta-1 and a 5' germline flanking sequence detects in EcoRI-digested DNA a 6.4-Kb germline fragment which carries D delta-3 and J delta-1 (fig. 2), and 3 additional bands of 3.0, 1.7 and 1.6-Kb. The latter fragments contain constant region sequences. The MH6 probe detects an 18-Kb germline fragment following BamHI digestion; this fragment contains D delta-3, J delta-1 and J delta-2. HindIII-

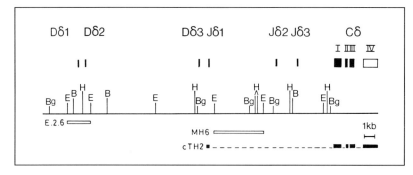

Fig. 1. Organization and partial restriction map of the TCR delta gene region. The probes used in the study are indicated below the map according to the source, i.e. genomic (open bars) or cDNA (closed bars). E, H, B, Bg denote EcoRI, HindIII, BamHI, and BglII restriction sites, respectively.

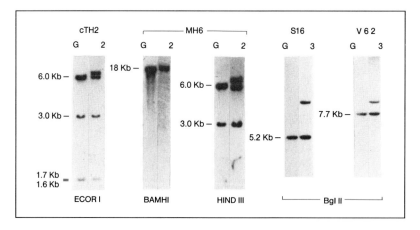

Fig. 2. Representative patterns od VDD rearrangement in ALL of infancy. Lane G shows the germline control. Lane numbers refer to individual patients.

cut germline DNA probed with MH6 produces a 6.0-Kb fragment containing D delta-3 and J delta-1 and a 3.0 fragment. However, the MH6 hybridizing sequences are 5' to J delta-2, and therefore MH6 can not detect rearrangements to this J. The S16 probe, as well as MH6, detects a 6.2-Kb BglII fragment that contains D delta-3 and J delta-1.

The E 2.6 probe is a 2.6-Kb EcoRI genomic fragment that contains D delta-1 and D delta-2 segments (all probes were kindly provided by Drs. T. Mak and M. Minden, Toronto, Canada, and Dr. T. H. Rabbits, Cambridge). The V delta-2 probe was isolated from a genomic library of a V delta-2 positive gamma/delta T-cell clone obtained from the PBL of a healthy donor [13].

The configuration of the TCR delta locus in ALL of infancy is summarized in table 1. Novel bands indicative of a TCR delta rearrangements were observed in 7 of the 20 cases (35 %). Deletion on one chromosome of C delta and J delta-3 coding sequences was found in one case (patient 19). Interestingly, two types of rearrangements accounted for all of the nondeletional delta locus involvements. The first one (observed in 5 of 7 cases) gave a characteristic pattern with the four restriction enzymes used: 19-Kb (BamHI), 6.4-Kb (EcoRI), 7.0-Kb (HindIII) and 9.9-Kb (BglII). Two samples showing this common type of rearrangement are reported in figure 2. In order to better characterize this type of rearrangement, we hybridized the same filters with a V delta-2 probe. As shown in the BglII-digests reported in figure 2, the V delta-2 detects the same 9.9-Kb fragment recognized by S16 (J delta-1). The evidences obtained using the different digestions strongly suggest that this type of rearrangement is due to an incomplete VDD joining.

The second pattern of rearrangement found (2 cases) is shown in figure 3. A fragment of 8.5-Kb (BglII) is characteristic of this pattern. After EcoRI and BamHI digestion, fragments of 3.5/3.8 and 10.5-kb were observed respectively (data not shown). In order to better clarify the nature of this rearrangement, we hybridized the same filter with the E 2.6 probe (figure 3). As shown in figure 3, for patient 11, the E 2.6 probe detects the same rearranged fragment recognized by the J delta 1 probe used (S16), strongly suggesting a DD 'partial' recombination on the basis of this second type of rearrangement.

The types of rearrangements observed in ALL of infancy are similar to the ones observed in B-cell precursor ALL of children [12]. The preference for incomplete attempts of V delta chain assembly is peculiar and contrasts with the results obtained in T-ALL (14). V delta-1 gene (which maps 5' to V delta-2) is more frequently involved in T-ALL and the rearrangements observed appear to be of V-(D)-J type, i.e. complete.

Conclusions

The analysis of Ig and TCR chain genes in ALL of infancy revealed some significant differences (incidence of multiple bands for Ig heavy-chain gene and TCR chain genes involvement) from ALL of children. These observations, in addition to the clinical (high WBC and poor response to treatment) and biological features (predominantly CD10 negative phenotype with a high frequency of myeloid antigen coexpression and chromosomal abnormalities involving band 11q23), confirm the unique feature of infant ALL when compared to ALL of children. Furthermore, the results of TCR delta chain gene configuration show that ALL of infancy to generally represent an earlier stage of lymphoid development than does ALL of other children.

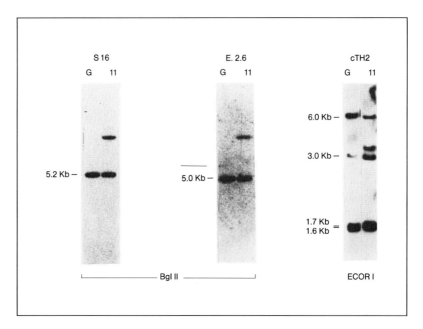

Fig. 3. Representative patterns of DD rearrangement in ALL of infancy. Lane G shows the germline control. Lane number refer to individual patients.

Summary

We analyzed Immunoglobulin (Ig) heavy chain, K light chain, and T-cell receptor (TCR) beta, gamma and delta TCR in 21 infant ALL cases. Each of these demonstrated leukemic cell surface antigens that were correlated with a B cell precursor phenotype. Ig heavy-chain gene rearrangements were detectable in all but one infant with leukemia. The analysis of Ig gene configuration revealed the presence of multiple rearranged fragments of variable autoradiographic intensities in 5 out of 21 (23 %) cases. In 3 infants we observed rearranged Ig K light-chain sequences. Rearrangements of TCR gamma and TCR beta occurred only in two patients and these findings are significantly different from those observed in B-cell precursor ALL of children. Novel bands indicative of TCR delta were observed in 7 out of 20 cases analyzed (35 %). Two patterns of TCR delta rearrangements were observed and both appeared to derive from partial joining: A VDD and a DD type. The results of TCR delta analysis seem to confirm that ALL of infancy generally represents an earlier stage of lymphoid development than does the ALL.

Acknowledgement

This work was partially supported by CNR, Progetto Finalizzato 'Biotecnologie e Biostrumentazione' (N.M.) and 'Oncologia' (R.F.), MPI 40 % (R.F.) and MPI 60 % (N.M. and R.F.). P.F.d.C. is a Ph.D. student in Experimental Hematology at the University of Milano. V.R is supported by Fondazione Tettamanti.

References

1 Reaman G, et al: Acute lymphoblastic leukemia in infants less than one year: A cumulative experience of the childrens cancer study group. J Clin Oncol 1985;3:1513.
2 Crist W, et al: Clinical and biological features predict a poor prognosis in acute lymphoid leukemias in infants: a pediatric oncology group study. Blood 1986;1:135.
3 Dinndorf PA, Reaman GH: Acute lymphoblastic leukemia in infancy: evidence for B cell origin of disease by use of monoclonal antibody phenotyping. Blood 1986;4:975.
4 Katz F, et al: Cellular and molecular studies on infant null acute lymphoplastic leukemia. Blood 1988;5:1438.
5 Pui CH, et al: An analysis of leukemic cell chromosomal features in infants. Blood 1987;5:1289.
6 Felix CA et al: Immunoglobulin and T cell receptor gene configuration in acute lymphoblastic leukemia of infancy. Blood 1987;70:536.
7 Rechavi G et al: More than two immunoglobulin heavy chain J region genes in the majority of infant leukemia. Leukemia 1988;6:347.
8 Brenner MB et al: The gamma/delta T cell receptor. Adv, Immunol 1988;43:133.
9 Chien YH, et al: T-cell receptor delta gene rearrangements in early thymocytes. Nature 1987;330:722.

10   Ludwig WD, et al: Phenotypic and genotypic heterogeneity in infant acute leukemia. I. Acute lymphoblastic leukemia. Leukemia 1989;3:431.

11   Waldmann TA: The arrangement of immunoglobulin and T-cell receptor genes in human lymphoproliferative disorders. Adv Immunol 1987;40:247.

12   Biondi A et al: High prevalence of T-cell receptor delta VDD or DD rearrangements in B-precursor acute lymphoblastic leukemias. Blood 1990;75:1834.

13   Casorati G et al: Molecular analysis of human gamma/delta[+] clones from thymus and peripheral blood. J Exp Med 1989;170:152.

14   Biondi A et al: T-cell receptor delta gene rearrangement in childhood T-cell acute lymphoblastic leukemia. Blood 1989;73:1989.

Dr. Andrea Biondi, Clinica Pediatrica, Ospedale San Gerardo,
Via Donizetti 106, I-20052 Monza (Italy)

Contrib Oncol. Basel, Karger, 1990, vol 41, pp 65–74.

Chromosomal Abnormalities
Involving the Short Arm of Chromosome 11
(Special Lecture)

T. Boehm, L. Foroni, J.M. Greenberg, A. Forster, I. Lavenir, T.H. Rabbitts

Medical Research Council Laboratory of Molecular Biology,
Cambridge, England

Zusammenfassung

Durch molekulargenetische Untersuchungen der Leukämiezellen von Patienten mit
T-ALL und der Translokation t(11;14) konnten die chromosomalen Bruchpunkte darge-
stellt werden, die den TCR δ-Genort auf Chromosomenband 14q11 betreffen, und eine
T-ALL «breakpoint cluster region» (bcr) auf dem kurzen Arm von Chromosom 11 bei 11p13
lokalisiert werden, nahe, aber mehr zentromer zum «Wilms-Tumor-Genort». Ein neues
Gen wurde bei einer Translokation t(11;14) (p15;q11) gefunden und charakterisiert. Da die-
ses neue 11p15 Gen unerwarteterweise im Zentralnervensystem anstatt im T-Zellsystem
exprimiert wird, könnte es sich um ein differenzierungs- statt proliferationsbezogenes
Onkogen handeln.

A number of consistent breakpoint clusters have been observed by
molecular cloning of DNA from human leukemias carrying chromosome
translocations. These include breaks near c-myc in Burkitt's lymphoma
[17], at the bcr locus in Philadelphia chromosome positive CML [13] and
ALL [16] and at the bcl-2 locus in follicular lymphoma [11]. In T-cell
tumours, the vast majority of chromosome abnormalities involve the T-cell
receptor δ/α locus at chromosome band 14q11 (reviewed [18]; [2]). In these
studies, three aspects of tumour-associated chromosomal observations can
be addressed. Firstly, these naturally occurring mutant chromosomes
should help to define the organisation of the human T-cell receptor δ/α
locus. Secondly, the mechanism by which chromosomal translocations/
inversions occur can be compared to the physiological assembly of variable

region genes via the VDJ-recombinase. Thirdly, the question can be asked as to whether a chromosomal aberration is crucial to tumour development. Here we briefly discuss these aspects with reference to two translocations involving two loci on the short arm of chromosome 11.

Results and Discussion

Chromosomal translocations involving the short arm of chromosome 11 establish the structure and location of the human TCR δ chain locus: Our detailed molecular study of a t(11;14)(p15;q11) translocation occurring in the RPMI8402 cell line identified a Jδ element as the translocation breakpoint on chromosome 14q11 and thereby established the spatial relationship of the human TCR δ locus to the TCR α locus chain gene [1, 4] (fig. 1). Further studies of t(11;14)(p13;q11) translocations established the location of D and J elements in the TCR δ chain locus [5] (fig. 1). The preponderance of breakpoints in the TCR δ chain locus in these immature T-cell tumours probably reflects the early rearrangements in this locus in T-cell ontogeny [8] and contrasts markedly with the location of breakpoints in the Jα region occurring in T-cell tumours of mature phenotype (fig. 1).

The structure of breakpoint junctions is equivalent to that of TCR δ chain variable region segments: Nucleotide sequence analyses obtained at the translocation junctions suggests that the inter-chromosomal exchange occurred during various stages of variable gene assembly. Table 1 exemplifies the extensive junctional diversification in the TCR δ chain variable-region by comparing the structure of a TCR δ chain cDNA clone (from IDP2) [15] to the $11p^+$ chromosomal junction of three translocation breakpoints [4, 5].

Translocations as errors of VDJ recombinase: Role of target sequences and chromosome accessibility: The involvement of recombinase by site-specific inter-chromosomal joining can be assessed by examination of sequences at translocation junctions. The VDJ recombinase recognises conserved heptamer/nonamer sequences for variable region gene assembly. Indeed, at some chromosomal junctions, signal-like sequences can be found [10] at the chromosomal locus not carrying an antigen receptor gene; however, others are clearly lacking such sequences [18].

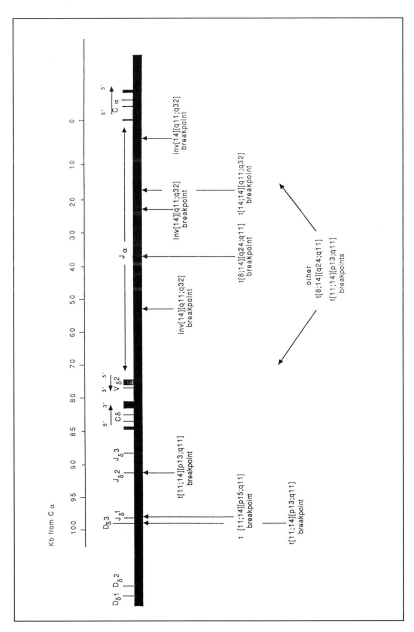

Fig. 1. The position of breakpoints of chromosomal aberrations involving the TCRδ/α locus. The organisation of TCR δ/α genes is indicated. The region between Vδ2 and Cα has many Jα elements [2].

Table 1. Junctional diversification in the T cell receptor δ chain

Source	5' element	N1	D δ 1	N2	D δ 2	N3	D δ 3	N4	3' element
IDP2	V δ 1	CTGTACGGG	GAAA	AC	TCCTA	GAAAGGAA	TGGGGGATACG	CGGTCTTTCCAT	J δ 1
LALW-2	11P13		AAT	CGGCAGG			CTGGGGGATACG		germ line sequences
RPMI8402	11P15			TGTGTCCCT	CTAC	CCAT	CTGGGGGATACG	TGGCGTACT	J δ 1
8511	11P13			GGTAGGATTACTTCC	TCCTAC	GG	CTGGGGA	CCTACGAGCCGCA	J δ 2
Germline			GAAATAGT		CCTTCCTAC		ACTGGGGGATACG		

These observations distinguish a two- and a one- site recognition model for sequence-specific recombinase involvement in these translocations [18]. The hypothesis of Alt and co-workers [20] suggests that prior transcription of elements to undergo rearrangement allows recombinase accessibility. However, in several well characterised translocations, no evidence for transcriptional activity near to the chromosomal breakpoints can be found [7]. In such cases, something intrinsic to the local DNA sequence at or near the translocation breakpoint may be important. One such putative sequence found near the junction of four different chromosomal abnormalities is a stretch of alternating purine/pyrimidine residues [7]; such potential Z-DNA stretches might allow perturbation of the chromatin in their locality, akin to transcription, thereby allowing recombinase access to the DNA. Thus rearrangement would be allowed merely as a consequence of DNA sequence and not by prior gene activity.

The T-ALL^{bcr} region is located near the Wilms' tumour predisposition locus and consistently disrupted in t(11;14)(p13;q11) translocations: The WT predisposition locus has been mapped to the short arm of chromosome 11 by virtue of consistent deletions in this chromosomal region in afflicted patients. The smallest region of overlap (S.R.O.) of these deletions define 11p13 as the site of this locus [19]. The spatial relationship of the T-ALL specific translocation breakpoint cluster region (T-ALL^{bcr}) to the WT predisposition locus was investigated [6]. The results indicated that the T-ALL^{bcr} lies very close to the WT locus (fig. 2a) [6]. A detailed restriction map of the T-ALL^{bcr} with the localisation of translocation breakpoints appears in figure 2b [5]. It is evident that the chromosomal breakpoints so far investigated all cluster within a very short region on chromosome 11p13. Indeed, our recent results suggest that 10 out of 10 breakpoints in t(11;14)(p13;q11) translocations can be mapped to the T-ALL^{bcr} region [12]. Several stretches of strong inter-species homology have been noted [7]. However, no gene has yet been found in this region; therefore, one has to consider several possibilities to explain the role of T-ALL^{bcr} in T-cell oncogenesis.

1. The T-ALL^{bcr} ist not transcribed, but exerts a regulatory influence on chromosome structure, etc., thereby influencing genes occurring at considerable distance from T-ALL^{bcr}. A precedent for this is the occurrence of variant breakpoints in Burkitt's lymphoma, which occur at distances greater than 100 kb from c-myc [3].

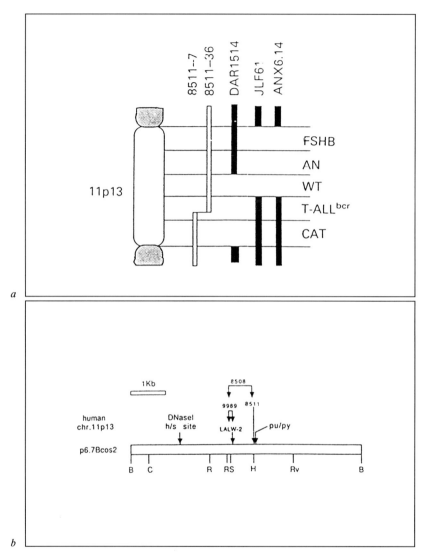

Fig. 2.a. Summary of somatic cell mapping data localising the T-ALL[bcr] region cen-tromeric to the position of the WT predisposition locus. Deletions observed in Wilms' tumour patients are schematically depicted (solid bars), whereas somatic cell hybrids made from a tumour with t(11;14)(p13;q11) translocation are indicated in open bars. Gene sym-bols are: FSHB, follicle stimulating hormone (β-subunit), AN, aniridia locus, WT, Wilms' tumour predisposition locus, T-ALL[bcr], breakpoint cluster region associated with t(11;14)(p13;q11) translocation, CAT catalase. (Adapted from [6]). *b.* Schematic representa-tion of the localisation of breakpoints on chromosome 11p13 [5].

2. The T-ALL[bcr] region actually belongs to a gene, the transcription of which is confined to a very small window in the cell cycle or ontogeny. Thus, the failure to find transcriptional activity is the consequence of this restricted pattern of expression.

Clearly, further studies are needed to distinguish between these possibilities.

Structure and expression characteristics of the gene found near a t(11;14) (p15;q11) breakpoint: We have previously observed transcriptional activity near a translocation junction in a rare chromosomal abnormality, namely t(11;14)(p15;q11) [4]. The structure of this gene in relation to the chromosomal translocation breakpoint has recently been elucidated [8], a summary of which appears in figure 3a. The gene is transcribed from two promoters; the alternative first exons each contain an AUG initiation codon and the protein is virtually identical irrespective of the promoter used. The predicted amino-acid sequence is highly conserved in evolution, a 98 % identity is observed between man and mouse (fig. 3b). The most intriguing aspect of the 11p15 gene, however, is the fact that a major site of expression is the central nervous system rather than T-cells [14]. Thus, the 11p15 gene could be an example of a differentiation-related oncogene (as opposed to oncogenes like c-myc, which are related to cell cycle control). The ectopic expression of a gene required in the central nervous system in T-cells induced by the translocation might thus be the tumorigenic event. In any case, with the elucidation of the gene structure, its role in T-cell tumorigenesis can now be directly assessed.

Summary

By examining leukemic cells of patients with T-ALL having the translocation t(11;14), the breakpoints of chromosomal aberrations involving the TCR δchain locus at chromosome band 14q11 was described, and a T-ALL breakpoint cluster region (bcr) was localized onto the short arm of chromosome 11 at 11p13, close but centromeric to the position of the Wilms' tumor predisposition locus. A new gene near a t(11;14)(p15;q11) breakpoint could be characterized, and as – unexpectedly – the central nervous system rather than the T-cell-system was found to be the site of expression, this 11p15 gene was supposed to be a differention- (rather than proliferation) related oncogene.

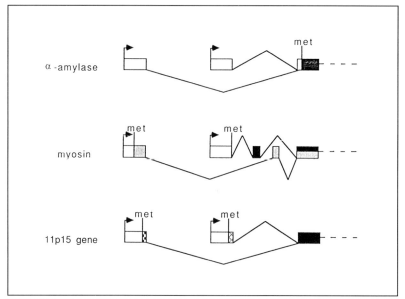

α-amylase

myosin

11p15 gene

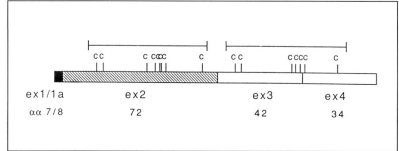

ex1/1a   ex2   ex3   ex4

αα 7/8   72   42   34

```
        EX 1/1A> <--- -------------------------- EX 2 -----------------------------------
HU1   MVLDQED GVPMLSVQPKGKQKGCAGCNRKIKDRYLLKALDKYWHEDCLKCACCDCRLGEVGSTLYTKANLIL
HU1A  M....K..^..................................................................
MO1   .......^..................................................................


        ------> <------------ EX 3 ------------------><--- EX 4 -
HU1   CRRDYLR LFGTTGNCAACSKLIPAFEMVMRARDNVYHLDCFACQLCNQR FCVGDKFFLKN
HU1A  .......^..............................^...........
MO1   .......^..............................^...........


        -----------------------------> 
HU1   NMILCQMDYEEGQLNGTFESQVQ
HU1A  .......................
MO1   ......V.....H..........

PROTEIN  WITH EX 1 = 155 AA, MW 17697
```

References

1   Baer R, Boehm T, Yssel H, Spits H, Rabbitts TH: Complex rearrangements within the human Jδ-Cδ/Jα-Cα locus and aberrant recombination between Jα segments. EMBO J 1988;7:1661–1668.

2   Boehm T, Rabbitts TH: The human T cell receptor genes are targets for chromosomal abnormalities in T cell tumours. FASEB J 1989;3:2344–2359.

3   Boehm T, Rabitts TH: A chromosomal basis of lymphoid malignancy in man. Eur J Biochem 1989;185:1–17.

4   Boehm T, Baer R, Lavenir I, Forster A, Waters JJ, Nacheva E, Rabbitts TH: The mechanism of chromosomal translocation t(11;14) involving the T-cell receptor Cδ locus on human chromosome 14q11 and a transcribed region of chromosome 11p15. EMBO J 1988;7:385–394.

5   Boehm T, Buluwela L, Williams D, White L, Rabbitts TH: A cluster of chromosome 11p13 translocations found via distinct D-D and D-D-J rearrangements of the human T cell receptor δ chain gene. EMBO J 1988;7:2011–2017.

6   Boehm T, Lavenir I, Forster A, Wadey RB, Cowell JK, Harbott J, Lampert F, Waters J, Sherrington P, Couillin P, Azoulay M, Junien C, van Heyningen V, Porteous DJ, Hastie ND, Rabbitts TH: The T-ALL specific t(11;14)(p13;q11) translocation breakpoint cluster region is located near to the Wilms' tumour predisposition locus. Oncogene 1988;3:691–695.

7   Boehm T, Mengle-Gaw L, Kees UR, Spurr N, Lavenir I, Forster A, Rabbitts TH: Alternating purine-pyrimidine tracts may promote chromosomal translocations seen in a variety of human lymphoid tumours. EMBO J 1989;8:2621–2631.

8   Boehm T, Greenberg JM, Buluwela L, Lavenir I, Forster A, Rabbitts TH: An unusual structure of a putative T cell oncogene which allows production of similar proteins from distinct mRNAs. EMBO J 1990;9:857–868.

Fig. 3. Structural comparison of the 11p15 gene and its protein products [8]. *a.* A diagrammatic comparison of the exon organisation of the 11p15, α-amylase and myosin genes. The various, relevant exons are indicated and the locations of the dual promoters in each gene are arrowed. The position within the gene of the methionine initiation codons are given (met) and the non-coding regions are as open boxes. RNA splicing alternatives are indicated. *b.* Diagrammatic representation of the 11p15 derived protein. The length of each exon in codons is shown with its delineation. The positions of cysteine residues within the putative protein are indicated and the apparently duplicated regions are overlined. *c.* Comparison of putative protein sequences derived from the two forms of human cDNA clones and the mouse clone. The full derived sequence, in the single letter code, is shown and the exon boundaries are indicated by arrow heads. Identity between residues in this sequences and the second human sequence or the mouse sequence are given as dots. (The exon boundaries of the mouse are not known because only cDNA sequence was obtained.)

9   Chien YH, Iwashima M, Kaplan KB, Elliott JF, Davis MM: A new T-cell receptor locus located within the alpha locus and expressed early in T-cell differentiation. Nature 1987;327:677–682.

10 Croce CM: Role of chromosome translocations in human neoplasia. Cell 1987;49:155–156.

11 Croce CM, Nowell PC: Molecular genetics of human B cell neoplasia. Adv Immunol 1987;38:245–274.

12 Foroni L, Boehm T, Lampert F, Kaneko Y, Raimondi S, Rabbitts TH: Multiple methylation-free islands flank a small breakpoint cluster region on 11p13 in the t(11;14)(p13;q11) translocation. Genes Chromosomes Cancer 1990;1:301–309.

13 Groffen J, Stephenson JR, Heisterkamp N, DeKlein A, Bartram CR, Grosveld G: Philadelphia chromosomal breakpoints are clustered within a limited region, bcr, on chromosome 22. Cell 1984;36:93–99.

14 Greenberg JM, Boehm T, Sofroniew MV, Keynes RJ, Barton SC, Norris ML, Surani MA, Spillantini MG, Rabbitts TH: Segmental and developmental regulation of a presumptive T-cell oncogene in the central nervous system. Nature 1990;344:158–160.

15 Hata S, Satyaniarayana K, Devlin P, Band H, McLean J, Strominger JL, Brenner MB, Krangel MS: Extensive junctional diversity of rearranged human T cell receptor δ genes. Science 1988;240:1541–1544.

16 Hermans A, Heisterkamp N, von Lindern M, Van Baal S, Meijer D, van der Plas D, Wiedemann LM, Groffen J, Bootsma D, Grosveld G: Unique fusion of bcr and c-abl genes in Philadelphia chromosome positive acute lymphoblastic leukemia. Cell 1987;51:33–40.

17 Rabbitts TH: The c-myc proto-oncogene: Involvement in chromosomal abnormalities. Trends Genet 1985;1:327–331.

18 Rabbitts RH, Boehm T, Mengle-Gaw L: Chromosomal abnormalities in lymphoid tumours: Mechanism and role in tumour pathogenesis. Trends Genet 1988; 4:300–304.

19 Riccardi VM, Hittner HM, Francke U, Yunis JJ, Ledbetter D, Borges W: The aniridia-Wilms' tumor association: the critical role of chromosome band 11p13. Cancer Genet Cytogenet 1980;2:131–137.

20 Yancopoulos GD, Alt FW: Developmentally controlled and tissue-specific expression of unrearranged VH segments. Cell 1985;40:271–281.

Thomas Boehm, Laboratory of Molecular Biology,
Hills Road, GB-Cambridge, CB2 2QH (UK)

Contrib Oncol. Basel, Karger, 1990, vol 41, pp 75–84.

Transient Myeloproliferative Disorders and Acute Leukemias in Infants with Down's Syndrome

U. Creutzig[a], *J. Ritter*[a], *J. Vormoor*[a], *C. Eschenbach*[b], *R. Dickerhoff*[c], *S. Burdach*[d], *H. G. Scheel-Walter*[e], *J. Kühl*[f], *G. Schellong*[a]

[a] Children's Hospital, University of Münster
[b] Children's Hospital, University of Marburg
[c] Children's Hospital, University of Bonn
[d] Children's Hospital, University of Düsseldorf
[e] Children's Hospital, University of Tübingen
[f] Children's Hospital, University of Würzburg, FRG

Zusammenfassung

Transiente, neonatale myeloproliferative Störungen (TMDs) wurden bei Neugeborenen mit Down-Syndrom beschrieben und können infolge Hepatosplenomegalie, Hautinfektionen, Leukozytose, Anämie, Thrombozytopenie nicht von akuter Leukämie unterschieden werden. Retrospektiv analysiert wurden 10 (unter 1 Jahr alte) aus einer Gesamtzahl von 30 Kindern mit Down-Syndrom und dem klinischen Bild einer AML oder myelodysplastischem Syndrom (MDS).

Bei allen 20 über 1 Jahr alten Kindern mit Down-Syndrom wurden eine akute myeloische Leukämie (AML) oder ein myelodysplastisches Syndrom (MDS) sicher diagnostiziert. Bei den 10 unter 1 Jahr alten Kindern wurde bei 3 eine Leukämieprogression mit Tod nach 2, 8 und 11 Monaten beobachtet. Bei den anderen 7 Säuglingen trat eine spontane (in einem Kind eine Interferon-induzierte) vollständige klinische und hämatologische Remission nach 4 bis 25 Wochen auf. Ein Patient zeigte eine zweite transiente leukämoide Reaktion 8 Monate später während einer Pneumonie. Bei allen außer den 3 Säuglingen mit echter Leukämie (im Alter von 1, 7 und 10 Monaten) konnte die Diagnose in den ersten Lebenstagen oder pränatal gestellt werden. Bei einem Kind wurde in der 35. Schwangerschaftswoche infolge Hydrops fetalis Fetalblut analysiert.

Durch die initialen klinischen und hämatologischen Befunde kann man nicht klar eine echte angeborene Leukämie von einer TMD unterscheiden. Eine Zuordnung von FAB-Subtypen durch morphologische, zytochemische und immunologische Kennzeichen bei TMD-Patienten war immer schwierig. Bei den meisten herrschten wenig differenzierte Blasten mit wenig oder keiner Zytoplasmagranulation vor, manchmal mit erythroblastären oder megakaryoblastären Ähnlichkeiten. Ein Patient zeigte morphologisch wie zytochemisch eine myelomonozytäre Differenzierung. Bei 3 Patienten zeigte die Immunphänotypanalyse Glycophorin A und/oder Megakaryozytenantigen-Expression bei geringer Expression von myeloischen Antigenen; bei 2 anderen Patienten waren die myeloischen Antigene vorherrschend.

Zur Unterscheidung von TDM von echter kongenitaler Leukämie sind am wichtigsten die zytogenetische Untersuchung des Leukämiekaryotyps und Stammzellkulturen. Im Zweifel, besonders bei Neugeborenen mit Down-Syndrom, sollte man mit der Chemotherapie solange abwarten, bis eine Progression zur Leukämie beobachtet wird oder bis zytogenetische Befunde die Leukämiediagnose erhärten können.

Down's syndrome is associated with a 10 to 20-fold increased incidence of acute lympho and myeloblastic leukemia (ALL and AML) compared to the general population [20, 22]. Other related hematological malignancies, such as preleukemic syndromes [27], acute myelofiobrosis [17], and non-Hodgkin's lymphoma [15] have also been described. In patients with Down's syndrome and AML, a high incidence of the otherwise extremely rare acute megakaryoblastic leukemia (FAB M7) has been reported [18, 25, 28, 30]. However, hematological disorders in patients with Down's syndrome often do not fit into standard classification systems.

Transient myeloproliferative disorders (TMD) have been observed mainly in neonates with Down's syndrome, and occasionally in phenotypically normal children with constitutional mosaicism of trisomy 21 [8].

In this retrospective analysis we compare the pretherapeutic characteristics and the outcome of patients with Down's syndrome and AML or myelodysplastic syndromes (MDS) with those having TMD during the first year of life.

Patients

From 1980–1989, 30 children with Down's syndrome and morphological and clinical features of AML or MDS of all age groups were reported to the AML study center in Münster. Three of these children at presentation had dysgranulo- and dyserythropoiesis in the bone marrow, but less than 30 % of blasts, and had to be classified as MDS. Twenty-seven were diagnosed as AML according to the FAB classification [2, 3].

The diagnosis TMD was based on the clinical observation of spontaneous remission within several weeks or months.

Children with Down's syndrome aged more than one year were excluded from this analysis. These children probably had true AML or MDS. Because most of them received chemotherapy, however, the diagnosis remains elusive. The diagnosis TMD was suggested in 7 out of 10 infants with Down's syndrome and clinical and morphological features of AML in the first year of life.

Results

Table 1 presents the initial clinical and hematological characteristics of the 10 children under one year of age with Down's syndrome and TMD or AML. The group of patients consisted of 8 boys and 2 girls. All TMD children were newborns in the first week of life, in contrast to children with true AML who were already 1, 7 or 10 months old at diagnosis. In one child (patient no. 3), fetal blood which was analyzed at the 35th week of gestation because of fetal hydrops showed undifferentiated blast cells, suggesting acute leukemia. At the time of birth, blood cell reduction had already occurred. Patient no. 1 had a second episode of TMD 8 months after the first one, along with severe pneumonia.

Hepatosplenomegaly was seen in most of the TMD cases as well as in the children with true leukemia. The hematological data varied in both groups of patients concerning leukocytosis, anemia and thrombocytopenia.

Morphologically, the blasts in TMD children (table 2) were mostly indistinguishable from poorly differentiated myeloblasts, often with

Table 1. Clinical and haematological data of under 1 year-old children with Down's syndrome and TMD or AML

Patient No.	Age (mo)	Sex	Liver (cm)	Spleen	Peripheral blood			
					WBC ($\times 10^3/mm^3$)	Blasts (%)	Platelets ($\times 10^3/mm^3$)	Hb (g/dl)
TMD patients								
1	(0) [+]	m	7	5	2.5	100	14	7.4
2	0	m	5	5	105	92	81	17.0
3	−0 [++]	f	?		176	53	110	12.8
4	0	f	3	0	73	42	364	14.8
5	0	m	3	5	50	57	91	11.6
6	0	m	3	1	64	44	175	21.3
7	0	m	5	4	17	41	40	13.0
AML patients								
8	1	m	0	0	40	75	?	?
9	7	m	2	6	13	40	16	13.8
10	10	m	2	0	5	0	16	7.6

[+] second episode of TMD 8 months later;
[++] prenatal diagnosis at the 35th week of gestation

erythroblastic and/or megakaryoblastic features with typical cytoplasmic budding. In patient no. 1, myelomonocytic differentiation was seen, with positive reaction of peroxidase (9 %) and the presence of a single Auer rod.

Immunological analysis revealed glycophorin A and/or megakaryocytic antigen expression, together with low expression of myeloid antigens in 3 children and predominant expression of myeloid antigens in another 2 children with TMD. In two of the AML children, myeloid antigens were present. However, definition of the FAB subtypes by morphological, cytochemical and immunological criteria was always difficult in TMD children as well as in the other children with Down's syndrome and true AML: The cytogenetic data only showed trisomy 21 and no additional abnormalities.

Table 3 shows the outcome in the TMD and AML patients with Down's syndrome. Two of the 3 infants with true AML were not treated, and died after 2 and 8 months following progression of leukemia. The third child was treated with α-interferon but also died due to progression of leukemia. In the 7 children with TMD, 1 child was treated with 6-thioguanine (2.5 mg/kg orally) for 8 weeks. In patient no. 7, the combination of α- and γ-interferon was given until SIDS occurred at the age of 11 months. There-

Table 2. Comparison of the morphological, immunological and cytogenetic data of children under 1 year of age with Down's syndrome and TMD or AML

Patients No.	Morphology		Immunology			Karyotype
	FAB	bone marrow blasts (%)	granulocytic antigens	erythroid antigens	megakaryocytic antigens	
TMD patients						
1	M4	74	+	−	−	+21
2	AUL	52	CD15 10%	Gly-A 50%	−	+21
3	AUL	24	−	Gly-A 18%	+	+21
4	(M7)	n.d.	CD33 50%	Gly-A 20%	gpIIb/IIIa 15%	
5	M1/6?	n.d.		Gly-A 4%		+21
6	AUL	100	CD33 55%	Gly-A 0%	−	+21
7	M6	44	CD15 +	Gly-A +	−	+21
AML patients						
8	M5a	61	+			+21
9	M6	15	incomprehensive			+21
10	M6	60	CD13/15/33 > 50%			+21

+ indicates presence of antigens without information about the percentage

Table 3. Outcome in children under 1 year of age with Down's syndrome and TMD or AML

Patients No.	Treatment	At discharge WBC (x10³/mm³)	blasts (%)	platelets (x10³/mm³)	Time until CR (weeks)	Survival (yrs / mos)	Cause of death
TMD patients							
1	(6-thioguanine)	2.1	0	53	8	5;10	—
2	—		no data		4	2;10	—
3	—	8.3	0	250	4	2;0	—
4	—	?	0	?	5	0;4	—
5	—	5–12	0	186	12–20	2;5	AML after 2 yrs!
6	—	2.5	0	24	> 17	6;1	—
7	α / γ -interferon	3.8	0	100	25	0;11	SIDS
AML patients							
8	—		—		progression	0;8	leukemia
9	—		—		progression	0;2	leukemia
10	α -interferon		12		partial remission	0;11	leukemia

fore, it is not possible to confirm the diagnosis TMD in this patient, as the remission was observed after interferon treatment. In 7 children, spontaneous (or interferon-induced) complete hematological recovery occurred within 4 and 25 weeks (median 8 weeks) from diagnosis. In 3 children, however, time until full hematological recovery (especially of the platelets) was 4–6 months. One of these children died of true AML developing 2 years later, after a preleukemic phase of 4 months. Morphologically and immunologically, this leukemia was classified as erythroleukemia (FAB M6).

Discussion

The results of our studies indicate that TMD is a phenomenon occurring mainly in neonatal or even prenatal life in children with Down's syndrome. The association of Down's syndrome with hematological malignancies has been documented for over 50 years [8]. Rosner et al. [22] described 22 (8 %) children with TMD among 276 children with Down's syndrome and clinical and hematological features of acute leukemia. In newborns, the percentage of TMD was almost 38 %, whereas Robison et al. [20] described no TMD among 115 children with Down's syndrome. Both authors reported a similar proportion of ALL vs. AML among children with Down's syndrome, compared with leukemic patients matched for age without Down's syndrome.

The morphological, immunological and clinical features of our TMD patients were indistinguishable from true AML or undifferentiated leukemia. In most cases the blasts were either unclassifiable (3 patients) or poorly differentiated, with some degree of erythroblastic or megakaryoblastic differentation (tab. 2). Recently, Cantù-Rajnoldi et al. [5] described leukemic reactions with megakaryocytic features in 5 newborns with Down's syndrome. Hayashi et al. [9] and Cook et al. [6] reported difficulties in classifying the blasts in these children.

The pathological mechanisms underlying the occurrence of acute leukemias and transient myeloproliferative disorders in children with Down's syndrome are unknown. A central role of the additional chromosome 21, has been suggested as trisomy 21 is also found in a considerable number of leukemic cell clones in constitutionally normal patients [1, 23]. An additional copy with consecutive dysregulation of genes on chromosome 21, which may be involved in hematopoietic cell proliferation (i.e. hu-ets-2), may therefore be suggested as the potential mechanism (gene dosage mechanism).

The transient myeloproliferative disorder seems to represent a non or premalignant state as indicated by the usually normal growth pattern of bone marrow cells in methyl-cellulose assays in patients with TMD [7, 12]. However, TMD may predispose to full malignant transformation, as suggested by the development of leukemia in children with prior transient leukemoid reactions (own observation – 1 patient [13, 14, 16, 31]). For full malignant transformation, additional genetic events seem therefore to be necessary. Accordingly, clonal chromosomal abnormalities other than trisomy 21, i.e. t(1;19) [16] or t(8;16) [19], could only be detected in patients with Down's syndrome and acute leukemia, and not in patients with TMD [9]. Some authors found a mixed growth pattern in stem cell cultures of patients with TMD, indicating the presence of an abnormal cell clone, which might have had already acquired additional genetic alterations, and possibly responsible for the development of AML at a later stage [31]. Further studies are necessary, however, to better understand the pathogenesis of TMD and acute leukemia in children with Down's syndrome.

TMD in phenotypically normal children is usually due to a mosaicism of trisomy 21 [4, 10, 26, 29]. In some cases, trisomy 21 may be confined to the expanding cell clone and no longer detectable in blood and tissue cells after spontaneous remission occurs [11, 24]. However, TMD very rarely has also been described in children without any detectable abnormality of chromosome 21 either in the tissue or blast cells [12].

For differential diagnosis of TMD and AML, a variety of disorders in the newborn period which can imitate leukemia have to be excluded: Congenital infection, hypoxemia and severe hemolysis are commonly associated with a leukemoid reaction. In addition, neonatal neuroblastoma may present hepatomegaly, subcutaneous nodules and bone marrow invasion, which may suggest congenital leukemia. The same occurs in histiocytosis X.

In the remaining children with Down's syndrome and the morphological picture of AML, we suggest applying cytogenetic analyses and stem cell cultures.

Concerning treatment, particularly in neonates with Down's syndrome, chemotherapy should be withheld for weeks or even months until definite progression of the leukemic process is observed or cytogenetic data indicating true leukemia are available.

Summary

Transient neonatal myeloproliferative disorders (TMDs), indistinguishable from acute leukaemia with hepatosplenomegaly, skin infiltration, peripheral leukocytosis, anaemia and thrombocytopenia have been described in neonates with Down's syndrome. To analyse the clinical significance of TMD, 10 infants (under 1 year of age) out of 30 children having Down's syndrome and the morphological picture of acute myelogenous leukaemia or myelodysplastic syndrome (MDS) were reviewed.

In all 20 children with Down's syndrome aged more than 1 year, the diagnosis of true AML or MDS was suggested. In 3 out of 10 infants, progression of leukaemia leading to death after 2, 8 and 11 months, respectively, was observed. In the other 7 infants, spontaneous (or in one child interferon-induced) complete clinical and haematological recovery occurred within 4 to 25 weeks of diagnosis. One of them had a second transient leukaemoid reaction 8 months later during a pneumonia. In all except the 3 infants with true leukaemia (aged 1, 7 and 10 months), diagnosis was made during the first days of life or prenatally. Fetal blood was analysed in one child at the 35th week of gestation because of fetal hydrops.

Initial clinical and haematological features did not allow differentiation of transient myeloproliferative disorders from true congenital leukaemia. However, definition of the FAB subtypes by morphological, cytochemical and immunological criteria was always difficult in TMD children. In most of the children, poorly differentiated blasts with few or no granulation were seen, sometimes with involvement of the nucleated red cell precursors and/or megakaryoblastic features. One child had morphological and cytochemical evidence of myelomonocytic differentiation. Immunological analysis revealed glycophorin A and/or megakaryocytic antigen expression together with low expression of myeloid antigens in 3 children and predominant expression of myeloid antigens in 2 other children.

Cytogenetic analyses and stem cell cultures may be useful in differentiating TMD from true congenital leukaemia. In cases of doubt, particularly in neonates with Down's syndrome, chemotherapy should be withheld until definite progression of the leukaemic process is observed or cytogenetic data indicating true leukaemia are available.

References

1   Allan RR, Wadsworth LD, Kalousek DK, Massing BG: Congenital erythroleukemia: A case report with morphological immunophenotypic, and cytogenetic findings. Am J Hematol 1989;31:114–121.

2   Bennett JM, Catovsky D, Daniel MT, Flandrin G, Galton DAG, Gralnick HR, Sultan C: Proposals for the classification of the acute leukaemias. Br J Haematol 1976;33:451–458.

3   Bennett JM, Catovsky D, Daniel MT, Flandrin G, Galton DAG, Gralnick HR, Sultan C: Criteria for the diagnosis of acute leukemia of megakaryocyte lineage (M7). Ann Intern Med 1985;103:460–462.

4   Brodeur GM, Dahl GV, Williams DL, Tipton RE, Kalwinsky DK: Transient leukemoid reaction and trisomy 21 mosaicism in phenotypically normal newborn. Blood 1980;55:691–693.

5   Cantu-Rajnoldi A, Cattoretti G, Caccamo ML, Biasini A, Bagnato L, Schiro R, Polli N: Leukaemoid reaction with megakaryocytic features in newborns with Down's syndrome. Eur J Haematol 1988;40:403–409.

6   Cook JA, Raney B, Innes DJ, Normanssell D: Transient myeloproliferative disorders, in a neonate with Down's syndrome, immunophenotypic studies. Clin Pediatr Phil 1989;28:132–135.

7   Denegri JF, Rogers PCJ, Chan KW, Sadoway J, Thomas JW: In vitro cell growth in neonates with Down's syndrome and transient myeloproliferative disorder. Blood 1981;58:675–677.

8   Fong CT, Brodeur GM: Down's syndrome and leukemia: epidemiology, genetics, cytogenetics and mechanisms of leukemogenesis. Cancer Genet, Cytogenet 1987;28:55–76.

9   Hayashi Y, Egushi M, Sugita K, Nakazawana S, Sato T, Kojima S, Bessho F, Konishi S, Inaba T, Hanada R et al: Cytogenetic findings and clinical features in acute leukemia and transient myeloproliferative disorder in Down's syndrome. Blood 1988;72:15–23.

10   Heaton DC, Fitzgerald PH, Fraser J, Abbott GD: Transient leukemoid proliferation of the cytogenetically unbalanced +21 line of a constitutional mosaic boy. Blood 1981;57:883–887.

11   Kalousek DK, Chan KW: Transient myeloproliferative disorder in chromosomally normal newborn infant. Med Pediatr Oncol 1987;15:38–41.

12   Lampkin BC, Peipon JJ, Price JK, Bove KE, Srivastava AK, Jones MM: Spontaneous remission of presumed congenital acute nonlymphoblastic leukemia (ANLL) in a karyotypically normal neonate. Am J Pediatr Hematol Oncol 1985;7:346–351.

13   Lazarus KH, Heerema NA, Palmer CG, Baehner RL: The myeloproliferative reaction in a child with Down's syndrome: Cytological and chromosomal evidence for a transient leukemia. Am J Hematol 1981;2:417–423.

14   Lin HP, Menaka H, Lim KH, Yong HS: Congenital leukemoid reaction followed by fatal leukemia: a case with Down's syndrome. Am J Dis Child 1980;134:939–941.

15   Lorenzana AN, Schorin MA: Non-Hodgkin's lymphoma in a neonate with Down's syndrome. Am J Pediatr Hematol Oncol 1989;11:186–190.

16   Morgan R, Hecht F, Cleary ML, Sklar J, Link MP: Leukemia with Down's syndrome: translocation between chromosomes 1 and 19 in acute myelomonocytic leukemia following transient congenital myeloproliferative syndrome. Blood 1985;66:1466–1468.

17   Pantazis CG, McKie VC, Sabio H, Davis PC, Allsbrook WC: Down's syndrome and acute myelofibrosis – Time study of DNA content during the progression to leukemia. Cancer 1988;61:2239–2243.

18   Peeters M, Poon A: Down syndrome and leukemia: Unusual clinical aspects and unexpected methotrexate sensitivity. Eur J Pediatr 1987;146:416–422.

19   Pettenati MJ, McNay JW, Chauvenet AR: Translocation of the mos gene in a rare t(8;16) associated with acute myeloblastic leukemia and Down's syndrome. Cancer Genet Cytogenet 1989;37:221–227.

20   Robison LL, Nesbit ME, Sather HN, Level C, Shahidi N, Kennedy A, Hammond D: Down syndrome and acute leukemia in children: A 10 year retrospective survey from the Children's Cancer Study Group. J Pediatr 1984;105:235–242.

21 Rogers PCJ, Thomas JW, Kalousek DK, Baker MA, Denegri JF: Neonate with Down's syndrome and transient congenital leukemia: In vitro studies. Am J Pediatr Hematol Oncol 1983;5:59–64.

22 Rosner F, Lee SL: Down's syndrome and acute leukemia: Myeloblastic or lymphoblastic. Am J Med 1972;53:203–218.

23 Rowley JD: Down syndrome and acute leukemia: Increased risk may be due to trisomy 21. Lancet 1981;II:1020–1022.

24 Sansone R, Haupt R, Strigini P, Garre ML, Panarello C, Cornaglia-Ferraris P: Congenital leukemia: Persistent spontaneous regression in a patient with an acquired abnormal karyotype. Acta Haematol 1989;81:48–50.

25 Sato T, Fuse A, Eguchi M, Hayashi Y, Ryo R, Adachi M, Kishimoto Y, Teramura M, Mizoguchi H, Shima Y, Komori I, Sunami S, Okimoto Y, Nakajima H: Establishment of a human leukaemic cell line (Cmk) with megakaryocytic characteristics from a Down's syndrome patient with acute megakaryoblastic leukemia: Br J Haematol 1989;72:184–190.

26 Seibel NL, Sommer A, Miser J: Transient neonatal leukemoid ractions in mosaic trisomy 21. J Pediatr 1984;104:251–254.

27 Sikand GS, Taysi K, Strandjord SE, Griffith R, Vietti TJ: Trisomy 21 in bone marrow cells of a patient with a prolonged preleukemic phase. Med Pediatr Oncol 1980;8:237–242.

28 Suarez CR, Le Beau MM, Silberman S, Fresco R, Rowley JD: Acute megakaryoblastic leukemia in Down's syndrome: Report of a case and review of cytogenetic findings. Med Pediatr Oncol 1985;13: 225–231.

29 Weinberg AG, Schiller G, Windmiller J: Neonatal leukemoid reaction: An isolated manifestation of mosaic trisomy 21. Am J Dis Child 1982;136:310–311.

30 Wilkie AOM, Kitchen C, Oakhill A, Howell RT, Berry PJ: Dicentric chromosome in the bone marrow of a child with megakaryoblastic leukaemia and Down's syndrome. J Clin Pathol 1988;41:378–380.

31 Wong KY, Jones MM, Srivastava AK, Gruppo RA: Transient myeloproliferative disorder and acute nonlymphoblastic leukemia in Down syndrome. J Pediatr 1988;112:18–22.

Priv.-Doz. Dr. Ursula Creutzig, Universitäts-Kinderklinik, Albert-Schweitzer-Str. 33, D-4400 Münster (FRG)

Contrib Oncol. Basel, Karger, 1990, vol 41, pp 85-86.

Transient Myeloproliferative Disorders (Abstract)

R. Sansone[a], S. Carobbi[a], M. Pierluigi[b], P. Strigini[a]

[a] Section of Epidemiological Genetics & Eco-Oncogenetics (EGEO)
National Cancer Institute, Genoa
[b] E.O. Galliera, Genoa, Italy

Congenital leukemia (CL) is still poorly understood and may in fact include a number of different hematologic disorders. Cases associated with Down's Syndrome (DS) not infrequently show a spontaneous regression [1]. Moreover, transient blastemia may be found also in phenotypically normal neonates with mosaic trisomy 21, presumably limited to hemopoietic system [2, 3]. Furthermore, some of the exceptional cases of transient non-DS-associated CL present clonal abnormalities involving chromosome 21 extracopies in leukemic cells [4]. Since in karyotypically normal leukemic neonates chemotherapy is usually started soon after diagnosis, the true figure of spontaneous remission in such cases is not known. These cases are probably rare events, even though some case reports have been published [5-7].

We would like to focus our attention on the following issues:

1) Pathogenesis of transient and non-transient CL in DS patients, in particular with respect to its peculiar association with the megakaryoblastic subtype (M7 FAB) [8, 9] and its possible origin through dysomic homozygosity in 21-trisomic cells [10];

2) Review of non-DS cases of transient CL;

3) Identification and evaluation of prognostic factors in CL to address a correct therapeutic protocol;

4) Comparison between transient myeloproliferative disorders in infants and transient remission (spontaneous or associated to exanguino-transfusion) of leukemia in other age group, through an analysis of old literature;

5) Leukemia cutis, with or without bone marrow involvement.

References

1 Engel RR, Hammond D, Eitzmann DV, Pearson H, Krivit W: Transient congenital leukemia in seven infants with mongolism. J Pediat 1964;65:303–305.

2 Brodeur GM, Dahl GV, Williams DL, Tipton RE, Kalwinsky DK: Transient leukemoid reaction and trisomy 21 mosaicism in a phenotypically normal newborn. Blood 1980;55:691–693.

3 Seibel NL, Sommer AM, Miser J: Transient neonatal leukemoid reaction in mosaic trisomy 21. J Pediatr 1984;104:251–254.

4 Van den Berghe H, Vermaelen K, Broeckaert-Van Orshoven A, Delbeke MJ, Benoit Y, Oryc E, Van Eygcn M, Logghe N: Pentasomy 21 characterizing spontaneously regressing congenital acute leukemia. Cancer Genet Cytogenet 1983;9:19–24.

5 Van Eys J, Flexner JM: Transient spontaneous remission in a case of untreated congenital leukemia. Am J Dis Child 1969;118:507–514.

6 Lampkin BC, Peipon JJ, Pice JK, Bove KE, Srivastava AK, Jones MM: Spontaneous remission of presumed congenital acute nonlymphoblastic leukemia in a karyotypically normal neonate. Am J Pediatr Hematol Oncol 1985;7:346–351.

7 Sansone R, Haupt R, Strigini P, Garre ML, Panarello C, Cornaglia-Ferraris P: Congenital leukemia: persistent spontaneous regression in a patient with an acquired abnormal karyotype. Acta Haematol 1989;81:48–50.

8 Lewis DS, Thompson M, Hudson E, Liberman MM, Samson D: Down's syndrome and acute magakaryoblastic leukemia: Case report and review of the literature. Acta Haematol 1983;70:236–242.

9 Suda J, Eguchi M, Ozawa T, Furukawa T, Hayashi Y, Kojima S, Maeda H, Tadokoro K, Sato Y, Miura Y, Ohara A, Suda T: Platelet peroxidase-positive blast cells in transient myeloproliferative disorder with Down's syndrome. Br J Haematol 1988;68:181–187.

10 Abe K, Kajii T, Niikawa N: Dysomic homozygosity in 21-trisomic cells: A mechanism responsible for transient myeloproliferative syndrome. Hum Genet 1989;82:-313–316.

Dr. Raffaele Sansone, Servizio di Epidemiologia,
Istituto Scientifico Tumori, Viale Benedetto XV, 10, I-16132 Genova (Italy)

Contrib Oncol. Basel, Karger, 1990, vol 41, pp 87–100.

Unusual Cytological Features of Hemoproliferative Disorders in the First Year of Life

A. Cantù-Rajnoldi[a], *P. Banfi*[a], *R. Schiró*[b], *L. Romitti*[c], *N. Polli*[d],
C. Valeggio[a], *M. Castagni*[a], *S. Pietri*[a], *A. Rovelli*[b], *G. Masera*[b]

[a] Laboratory of Clinical Research, Clinical Institute 'Perfezionamento', Milan
[b] Department of Pediatrics, University of Milano, E.O.G., Monza
[c] Divison of Cytogenetics, Clinical Institute 'Perfezionamento', Milan
[d] National Tumor Institute, Milan, Italy

Zusammenfassung

Hämoproliferative Störungen können im ersten Lebensjahr zytologisch ungewöhnlich aussehen. Unsere Erfahrungen zwischen 1982 und 1989 beziehen sich auf folgende hämoproliferative Störungen: a) Megakaryozytäre leukämoide Reaktion bei Säuglingen mit Down-Syndrom; b) akute undifferenzierte Leukämie; c) akute Leukämie mit gemischt myeloischen und monozytären Zügen.

a) 5 Neugeborene/Säuglinge mit Down-Syndrom zeigten eine leukämoide Reaktion, gekennzeichnet durch vorherrschende Blasten megakaryozytärer Herkunft. Die Blastenpopulation wurde in jedem Fall durch Immunphänotypisierung und in 2 Fällen auch durch die Plättchen-Peroxydasereaktion untersucht. Eine Spontanremission trat immer nach wenigen Wochen ein. In einem Fall wurde jedoch nach 16 Monaten ein Rezidiv der myeloproliferativen Störung diagnostiziert, aber mit niedrig-dosiertem ARA-C wieder in Vollremission gebracht.

b) Die akute undifferenzierte Leukämie (AUL), häufig verbunden mit Hyperleukozytose und schlechter Prognose, ist im 1. Lebensjahr vorherrschend. Die zellmorphologischen Untersuchungen bei unseren Patienten wiesen Besonderheiten auf wie einen gewissen Dimorphismus der Blasten. In einem Fall trat eine ausgeprägte Hyperleukozytose mit monozytären Zügen 1 Woche nach der Diagnose einer t(4;11)-AUL auf, was als Zielzelle der leukämischen Transformation in diesem Falle eine gemeinsame lympho-monozytäre Vorläuferzelle nahelegt.

c) Bei 3 Patienten waren die morphologischen und zytochemischen Befunde inkompatibel mit den FAB-Kriterien der akuten myeloischen Leukämie und deuteten daher auf eine gemischte myelo-monozytäre Herkunft. In diesen Fällen zeigte die Blastenpopulation viele Zytoplasmagranula und starke Myeloperoxidase-Positivität. Die unspezifischen Esterasen waren jedoch bei den meisten Zellen stark positiv. Weiter konnten spezifische myeloische und monozytäre Antigene durch Immunphänotypisierung nachgewiesen werden. Bei allen 3 Patienten war die ausgeprägte Hyperleukozytose mit schlechter Prognose einhergehend.

Some hematological disorders or malignancies may present unusual features in the first year of life; their incidence is unusually high. A well-known example of this is the leukemoid reaction in newborns with Down's syndrome, which apparently depends on transient abnormal myelopoiesis [19]. Patients with Down's syndrome also have an abnormally high risk of developing acute leukemia [15, 18, 22], and acute megakaryoblastic leukemia is frequently associated with Down's syndrome (Lewis et al. 1983; Bevan et al. 1982; Cairney et al. 1985) [4, 5, 17]. In this paper we describe five newborns/infants with Down's syndrome who developed a transient leukemoid reaction in which a high percentage of blast cells belonging to the megakaryocytic series was observed in the peripheral blood and bone marrow. We also describe our experience of acute leukemia in infants, which confirms the high incidence of acute unidfferentiated leukemia (AUL) [9]. In one such case with a t(4;11), a striking shift of phenotype, from lymphoid to monocytoid, was observed a week after the start of treatment. Finally, an unusual non-promyelocytic hypergranular type of acute non-lymphoid leukemia (ANLL) characterized by the cytochemical and immunological coexpression of monocytic and granulocytic features was observed in two children. A two year old child affected by the same disorder with strong clinical and biological similarities with the other two cases is also described.

Materials and Methods

Peripheral blood and bone marrow samples from different institutions were all studied at the Laboratorio di Ricerche Cliniche, Istituti Clinici di Perfezionamento in Milan. The smears were stained with May-Grunwald Giemsa and the cytochemical stains performed according to Shibata et al. [21]. The immunophenotype was determined by immunocytochemical reactions (immunoperoxidase using the avidin-biotin complex (ABC) technique or the alkaline phosphatase anti-alkaline phosphatase (APAAP) technique) on smears or cytocentrifuged cells, or on mononuculear cells separated by Ficoll-Hypaque density gradient and stained for indirect immunofluorescence evaluation under the fluorescence microscope.

The monoclonal antibodies (MAbs) used were J5 (CD10), B4 (CD19), OKB2 (CD24), BA-2 (CD9), WT1 (CD7), T1 (CD5), T3 (CD3), OKM1 (CD11b), My7 (CD13), My4 (CD14), LeuM1 (CD15), My9 (CD33), FMC25 (CD42a), C17.27 (CD41), 7.2 (MHC class II). Terminal transferase (TdT) was determined using polyclonal antibodies (Hybritech) or

MAbs (Technogenetics) by indirect immunofluorescence or immunocytochemical techniques.

For transmission electron microscopy (TEM) analysis, cells were fixed in 3 % glutaraldehyde in 0.1 mol/1 phosphate buffer at pH 7.0 for 1 h, post-fixed in 1 % osmium tetroxide and stained with uranyl acetate. They were then embedded in 3 % agar, dehydrated and embedded in Araldite. Thin sections were stained with 5 % uranyl acetate in ethanol and Reynold's lead citrate and viewed under a Philips 410 TEM. The platelet peroxidase reaction (PPO) was performed according to the method of Roels et al. [20].

Cytogenetic analysis was performed on bone marrow samples (either by a direct method and/or after culture for 24 h) and/or unstimulated blood cells cultured for 24 h. Chromosomes were analyzed with the Q-banding method.

Results

Megakaryocytic leukemoid reaction in newborns/infants with Down's syndrome: Main clinical and hematological data in five newborns/infants with Down's syndrome and a megakaryocytic leukemoid reaction are listed in table 1. Age ranged from 1 day to 2 months; anemia was present in one case and mild to severe thrombocytopenia in four. WBC counts ranged from 25.0×10^3 to 95.4×10^3 and the blast percentage in the peripheral blood from 33 to 72 %. The leukemoid picture regressed spontaneously in all five patients after 5 – 13 weeks. However, in one patient (C. E.), a relapse of the myeloproliferative disorder occurred after 16 months and the blast cell population showed the same characteristics as previously. The child was treated with low-dose Ara-C (20 mg/m^2/d i. v.) for 21 days because of the relevant clinical involvement. The clinical and the hematological picture regressed and the child was placed in maintenance therapy for 18 months, with monthly cycles of of low-dose Ara-C; she was off therapy and in complete remission at 39 months of age.

Table 1. Main clinical and laboratory data in newborns/infants with Down's syndrome

Case	Age	Hb g/dl	WBC x 10^3	Blasts % PB	Plts x 10^3	Outcome
N.G.	10 days	15.5	25.0	42	265	remission after 10 weeks
B.M.	1 day	17.0	78.0	37	30	remission after 8 weeks
C.E.	2 days	19.0	69.0	63	29	remission after 13 weeks*
D.V.	2 months	6.9	95.4	72	103	remission after 5 weeks
S.T.	9 days	18.9	35.0	33	55	remission after 6 weeks

* Relapse at 19 months. CR was then obtained with LD Ara-C

Morphology at light microscopy was characterized by a certain heterogeneity of the blast cells; however, in all cases some cells showed features suggesting a megakaryocytic origin as irregular cytoplasmic projections, hyperchromic naked nuclei and fine azurophilic granules (fig. 1). Positive reactions for acid phosphatase (AcP) and alpha-naphthyl-acetate esterase (ANAE) were often observed; alpha-naphthyl-butyrate esterase was always negative, and PAS positive blocks or granules were sometimes seen.

The immunophenotype showed a clear positivity for the anti-megakaryocytic MAbs in a considerable part of blasts (fig. 2), whereas the anti-T, anti-B and anti-myeloid MAbs were unreactive. Cytochemical and immunological data are summarized in table 2.

Ultrastructural morphology and cytochemistry were performed in cases 1 and 2. Cells with megakaryoblastic features (high N/C ratio, evident nucleolus, no cytoplasmic differentiation features except for some strands of endoplasmic reticulum, sometimes rare granules and a PPO positivity restricted to the perinuclear membrane and endoplasmic reticulum) were identified together with blasts showing a myeloid differentiation (more abundant cytoplasm, better developed endoplasmic reticulum, numerous

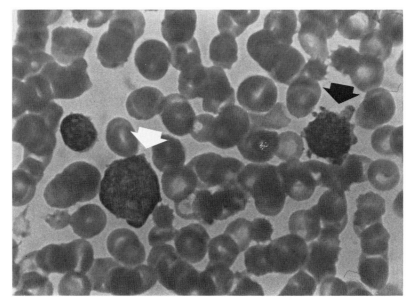

Fig. 1. Leukemoid reaction in newborns with Down's syndrome: A micromegakaryoblast (black arrow) with an undifferentiated blast (white arrow) and a lymphocyte (peripheral blood, MGG x 1,000).

cytoplasmic granules and a PPO reaction were also present in the granules and Golgi area).

Acute undifferentiated leukemia: AUL is defined as non-T, non-B, CD10⁻, light microscopy MPO⁻ acute leukemia, in which acute monocytic leukemia was also excluded for the absence of the needed morphological and cytochemical criteria according to the FAB classification [1]. AUL is particularly common in the first year of life; eleven of 27 cases (40.7 %) of

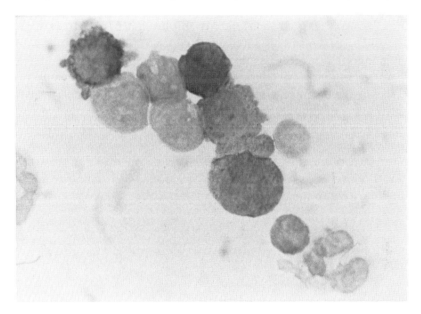

Fig. 2. Leukemoid reaction in newborns with Down's syndrome. C17.27 (CD41) reactivity on peripheral blood blast cells (APAAP technique x 1,000).

Table 2. Immunological and cytochemical data in newborns/infants with Down's syndrome

Case	CD10	HLA-DR %	TdT	CD41 %	CD42a %	CD7	CD11b	ANAE %	AcP %
N.G.	neg	10	neg	46	49	neg	neg	70 foc	80 diff
B.M.	neg	12	neg	60	60	neg	neg	75 foc	66 foc
C.E.	neg	3	neg	18	51	neg	neg	90 diff	33 foc
D.V.	neg	2	neg	30	30	neg	neg	10 foc	70 foc
S.T.	neg	9	neg	23	nt	neg	neg	80 foc	90 gran/foc

diff: diffused; foc: focal; gran: granular; nt: not tested

acute leukemia diagnosed in infants at our Institutions presented these characteristics. Morphology of the blast cell populations frequently showed a highly immature nuclear chromatin. Cellular dimorphism, with cells presenting monocytoid features together with more undifferentiated cells, was often seen (fig. 3). A high incidence of ANAE positivity was also noted (5 of 10 cases tested). Common features were hyperleukocytosis (mean WBC count: 413.9×10^3/mmc) and coexpression of one or more myeloid antigens (CD11b, CD13, CD14, CD 15, CD33) with B-lymphoid antigens (CD19, CD24, CD9) in six of nine cases tested for at least two anti-myeloid MAbs. TdT was positive in 9 of 11 cases. A striking peripheral monocytosis (WBC 26.3×10^3 with 72 % of monocytoid cells), which regressed progressively in a few days (fig. 4), was observed in one of these cases (M. S.) after seven days of therapy.

The main clinical and cytogenetic data are listed in table 3, and cytochemical and immunological data in table 4. Of the eight cases tested, four presented a t(4;11), one a t(x;10)(p11;p11) and three had a normal karyotype.

Acute non-lymphoid leukemia with mixed myeloid and monocytic features: Three patients aged six, five and twenty-four months respectively presented a morphological picture characterized by atypical myeloid blasts

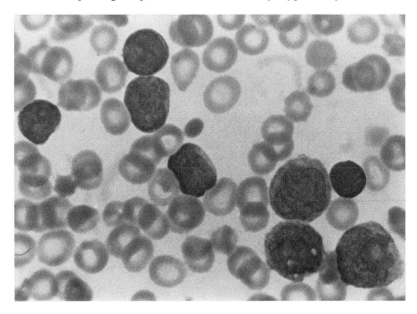

Fig. 3. Acute Undifferentiated leukemia: Undifferentiated and monocytoid blasts in the peripheral blood (MGG x 1,000).

with a hypergranular cytoplasm and no Auer rods (fig. 5). The overall aspect differed from that of a typical promyelocytic leukemia in the absence of Auer rods, and the larger sizes and less clumped arrangement of the granules. Myeloperoxidase (MPO) was strongly positive in the great majority of

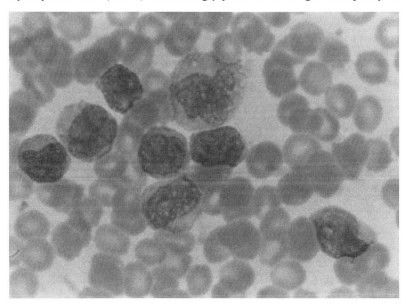

Fig. 4. Acute undifferentiated leukemia: Peripheral blood monocytosis in a patient with a t(4;11) seven days after starting chemotherapy (MGG x1,000).

Table 3. Clinical and cytogenetic data in infants with acute undifferentiated leukemia

Case	Age mths	WBC x 10^3	Karyotype	Clinical outcome
G.R.	5	?	t(4;11)	lost at the follow up
I.G.	4	424	t(4;11)	therapy resistant
L.D.	5	500	t(4;11)	BM relapse after 11 months
M.S.	1	790	t(4;11)	CCR
B.M.	4	26.8	t(xp;10p)	CCR
Y.A.	9	756	46, xx	BM relapse after 11 months
D.U.	7	200	46, xy	BM relapse after 17 months
B.C.	3	940	46, xx	died in the induction phase
D.M.	1	57	not tested	died in the induction phase
S.M.	10	59.5	not tested	in therapy (induction)
P.D.	4	386	not tested	in therapy (induction)

Table 4. Cytochemical and immunological data in infants with acute undifferentiated leukemia

Case	PAS %	ANAE %	AcP %	TdT	B-markers			Myeloid markers				
					CD19	CD24	CD9	CD33	CD15	CD11b	CD13	CD14
G.R.	65	70	−	+	+	−	+	−	+	−	+	−
I.G.	69	nt	nt	+	nt	−	−	nt	nt	−	nt	nt
L.D.	−	−	−	+	+	+	−	nt	−	−	−	−
M.S.	25	−	−	+	+	−	+	+	−	−	−	nt
B.M.	60	−	−	+	nt	nt	nt	nt	nt	nt	nt	nt
Y.A.	−	90	−	+	+	+	+	−	+	−	−	−
D.U.	−	−	−	+	+	+	+	−	−	−	−	nt
B.C.	58	44	−	−	+	−	+	−	+	nt	−	−
D.M.	14	15	14	+	+	+	+	+	+	+	+	+
S.M.	−	20	90	−	−	−	−	+	−	nt	−	−
P.D.	56	−	−	+	+	−	nt	−	−	−	−	−

TdT+: ≥ 10 %; Other MoAbs+: ≥ 20 %; nt: not tested

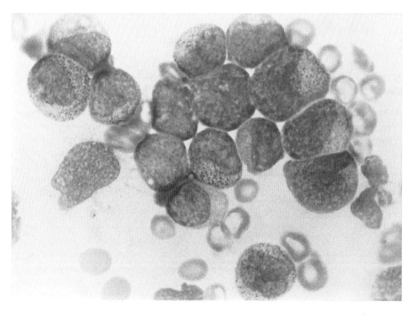

Fig. 5. Acute non lymphoid leukemia with mixed myeloid and monocytic features: hypergranular non-promyelocytic blasts in the bone marrow (MGG x 1,000).

blasts, as were ANAE. The myeloid esterases (chloro-acetate esterase, CAE) were coexpressed in a varying number of cells. The immunophenotype of all three cases presented some degree of reactivity for monocytic MAbs (CD14) as well for other myeloid MAbs (CD11b, CD15 and CD33). HLA-DR was absent or expressed in a low percentage of blasts.

Cytogenetic analysis revealed a normal karyotype in one patient (A. J.) and an involvement of chromosome 11 in two patients (A. E. and V. D.), the former presenting a t(5;11)(q21;q24) and the latter a del(11)(q21q23).

Clinically, these cases were characterized by a marked hyperleukocytosis, overt bleeding and laboratory evidence of disseminated intravascular coagulation (DIC) in two cases (A. E. and V. D.), and a fatal outcome, one (A. E.) being resistant to chemotherapy and the other two relapsing a few months later. Survival was 13 months (A. J.), two months (A. E.), and 8 months (V. D.). The main clinical and laboratory data of these three patients are summarized in tables 5 and 6.

Table 5. Clinical and cytogenetic data in infants with atypical acute non-lymphoblastic leukemia

Case	Age (months)	WBC (x 10^3)	Karyotype	Outcome	Survival (months)
A.J.	6	147	46,xy	CNS relapse after 7 months	13
A.E.	5	540	46,xx,t(5;11)(q21;24)	No CR	2
V.D.	24	192	46,xy, del(11)(q21q23)	BM relapse after 5 months	8

Table 6. Main cytochemical and immunological data in infants with atypical acute non-lymphoblastic leukemia

Case	Cytochemistry (%)				HLA-DR %	My Mabs
	MPO	ANAE	CAE	AcP		
A.J.	74	99	30	90	8	CD11b = 48 % CD14 = 35 %
A.E.	88	90	70	neg	12	CD11b = 38 % CD14 = 39 %
V.D.	95	98	90	95	30	CD11b = 37 % CD14 = 22 % CD15 = 45 % CD33 = 90 %

Discussion

This paper reports our experience of some hematological disorders with unusual features present in the first year of life. First, we described five newborns with Down's syndrome, three of them previously reported [6], showing a leukemoid reaction characterized by a considerable percentage of the blast cells being megakaryocytic precursors. A similar hematological picture was described by Coulombel et al. [8] and by Bessho et al. [3] respectively in two and five newborns with Down's syndrome. The presence of blasts with a myeloid distribution of the PPO reaction in one of our cases and in all the cases described by Bessho et al. [3] and Coulombel et al. [8] provided clear evidence that blasts belonging to other hematopoietic cell lineages were involved in addition to megakaryoblasts. Moreover, a PPO distribution in polyribosomes [3] and the presence of ferritin molecules at ultrastructural level [8] suggested the erythroid origin of some blasts. Three of the patients described by Bessho et al. died in a few weeks from pneumonia, DIC and heart failure, respectively, and cannot be analyzed in a followup of the leukemoid reaction, even though in one of them the blasts had already disappeared from the peripheral blood. A spontaneous regression of the leukemoid picture was observed in the other nine patients reported in the literature and in the present series. Nevertheless, in one of our cases and in one each of those described by Bessho et al. and Coulombel et al., the leukemoid picture recurred some months later. Low-dose Ara-C was given in our case and the hematological picture normalized again, whereas no improvement was reported by Coulombel et al. and no further details were given by Bessho et al. The benign or neoplastic nature of this transient myeloproliferative disorder is still unclear in the absence of a definite clonal marker for these cells. However, a neoplastic condition should be at least suspected in some of these cases because of the possibility of reappearance of blast cells some months later and/or the coexistence of additional chromosomal abnormalities [8].

We also presented our data on eleven cases with AUL, emphasizing the frequent presence of blasts with morphologic monocytoid features together with lymphoid or more undifferentiated blasts, the high incidence of coexpression of B-related antigens and myeloid-monocytic antigens, and the unusual high percentage of ANAE positivity. Coexpression of myeloid antigens was detected in six of nine cases tested for at least two anti-myeloid MAbs; CD15 positivity was found in four cases, CD33 in three, CD13 in two, CD11b and CD14 in one. These data suggest a derivation of the leukemic clone from a common lympho-myelo-monocytic precursor. The shift observed in vivo in one of our cases from an undifferentiated phenotype to an overt monocytoid phenotype clearly strengthens this hypothesis although the biological mechanism underlying this phenomenon needs to be clarified. A similar effect both in vitro and in vivo has been observed in a neonatal acute leukemia with a t(4;11) by using deferoxamine [11]. The use of agents promoting cellular differentiation that may be combined with chemotherapy for treatment of this type of leukemia should be investigated in the future, also in light of the usually very bad prognosis observed in these cases. It is stressed that the incidence of karyotype abnormalities involving the 11q23 region, particularly a t(4;11), is high, in agreement with reports in the literature of the last years [12–14].

Finally, we described three patients, two of them briefly presented elsewhere [7], with an unusual type of ANLL, not classifiable according to the FAB classification [1], showing a mixture of monocytic (ANAE and CD14 positivity) and granulocytic features (hypergranular cytoplasm, MPO and CAE positivity). Acute promyelocytic leukemia (APL) presents some similarities such as hypergranular cytoplasm, strong MPO positivity, and characteristic HLA-DR negativity [10]. Moreover, some monocytic features as a certain degree of ANAE positivity [23], as well as CD14 positivity [10] are fequently found in APL. Nevertheless, in addition to some cytological differences (absence of Auer rods and a less clumped arrangement of the granules), we did not observe a t(15;17) in these cases which is closely and non-randomly associated with APL [16]. On the contrary, in two of three cases we found anomalies involving chromosome 11, a t(5;11)(q21;q24) and a partial deletion (q21q23). It is well known that chromosome 11 abnormalities are often associated with monocytic variants of ANLL [2]. A t(5;11) has been described in two cases of myelomonocytic leukemia [2, 24], and a del(11) with breakpoints similar to that shown in our case has also been observed in cases of acute monocytic leukemia [2, 24]. In conclusion, this ANLL variant, which we have only diagnosed in children under two years, has some features in common with both APL and acute monocytic leukemia, and probably originates from a progenitor at an intermediate promyelocytic-monocytic stage of differentiation.

Summary

Some hematological disorders may present unusual features in the first year of life. We describe our experience of the following hemoproliferative disorders in the period

1982–1989: a) Megakaryocytic leukemoid reaction in infants with Down's syndrome; b) acute undifferentiated leukemia; c) acute leukemia with mixed myeloid and monocytic features.

a) We observed five newborns/infants with Down's syndrome who presented a leukemoid reaction characterized by the prevalence of blast cells of the megakaryocytic lineage. In each case, the blast cell population was studied by immunophenotyping, and in two cases also by the platelet-peroxidase reaction. A spontaneous remission always occurred in a few weeks. However, in one case, a relapse of the myeloproliferative disorder was diagnosed 16 months later and a complete remission then achieved with low-dose Ara-C.

b) Acute undifferentiated leukemia (AUL) is common in the first year of life and is frequently associated with hyperleukocytosis and a poor clinical outcome. In our patients, morphological investigations showed some unusual characteristics, such as a certain dimorphism of the blast cells. In one case a marked hyperleukocytosis with monocytoid features occurred a week after a diagnosis of AUL associated with a t(4;11), further suggesting that a common lympho-myelomonocytic precursor is the target of leukemic transformation in this kind of leukemia.

c) Morphogical and cytochemical features incompatible with the FAB criteria for the diagnosis of acute myeloid leukemia and indicating a mixed myeloid-monocytic origin were observed in three patients. In these cases, the blast cell population showed many cytoplasmic granules and strong myeloperoxidase positivity. However, unspecific esterases were highly positive in the majority of cells. Specific myeloid and monocytic antigens were detected by immunophenotyping. A striking hyperleukocytosis was associated with poor outcome in all 3 patients.

Acknowledgements

We wish to thank Dr. G. Cattoretti (Istituto Nazionale Tumori, Milan, Italy) for his critical reading of the manuscript and Dr. A. Biasini (Ospedale M. Bufalini, Cesena, Italy) for co-operation in the diagnosis of one of the patients with Down's syndrome. Financial support was given by: Regione Lombardia, Progetto di Ricerca finalizzata (L. R. 31. 8. 1981) per l'area 'Diagnosi e Terapia'.

References

1   Bennett JM, Catovsky D, Daniel MT, Flandrin G, Galton DAG, Gralnick HR, Sultan C: Proposed revised criteria for the classification of acute myeloid leukemia. Ann Intern Med 1985;103:626–629.

2   Berger R, Flandrin G, Bernheim A, Le Coniat M, Vecchione D, Pacot A, Derré J, Daniel MT, Valensi F, Sigaux F, Ochoa-Nogerua ME: Cytogenetic studies on 519 consecutive de novo acute nonlymphocytic leukemias. Cancer Genet Cytogenet 1987;29:9–21.

3   Bessho F, Hayashi Y, Hayashi Y, Ohga K: Ultrastructural studies of peripheral blood of neonates with Down's syndrome and transient abnormal myelopoiesis. Am J Clin Pathol 1988;89:627–633.

4   Bevan D, Rose M, Greaves MF: Leukaemia of platelet precursors: Diverse features in four cases. Br J Haematol 1982;51:147–164.

5   Cairney AEL, Mc Kenna R, Arthur DC, Nesbit ME jr. Woold WG: Acute megakaryo-blastic leukaemia in children. Br J Haematol 1985;63:541–554.

6   Cantù-Rajnoldi A, Cattoreti G, Caccamo ML, Biasini A, Bagnato L, Schirò R, Polli N: Leukaemoid reaction with megakaryocytic features in newborns with Down's syndrome. Eur J Haematol 1988;40:403–409.

7   Cattoretti G, Delia D, Parola L, Schirò R, Valeggio C, Simoni G, Romitti L, Polli N, Lambertenghi-Deliliers G, Ferrari M, Cantù-Rajnoldi A: Heterogenous expression of myelomonocytic markers on selected non-lymphoid cells, in Leukocyte typing II: Human myeloid and hematopoietic cells. Berlin, Springer 1986, pp 217–235.

8   Coulombel L, Derycke M, Villeval L, Loenard C, Breton-Gorius J, Vial M, Bourgeois P, Tchernia G: Characterization of the blast cell population in two neonates with Down's syndrome and transient myeloproliferative disorder. Br J Haematol 1987;66:69–76.

9   Crist W, Pullen J, Boyett J, Falletta J, van Eys J, Borowitz M, Jackson J, Dowell B, Frankel L, Quddus F, Ragab A, Vietti T: Clinical and biologic features predict a poor prognosis in acute lymphoid leukemias in infants: A pediatric oncology group study. Blood 1986;67:135–140.

10 Das Gupta A, Sapre RS, Shah A, Advani SH, Nair CH: Cytochemical and immuno-phenotypic heterogeneity in acute promyelocytic leukemia. Acta Haematol 1989;81:5–9.

11 Estrov Z, Tawa A, Wang X, Dubé ID, Sulh H, Cohen A, Gelfand EW, Freedman H: In vitro and in vivo effects of deferoxamine in neonatal acute leukemia. Blood 1987;69:757–761.

12 Hagemeijer A, van Dongen JJM; Slater RM, van't Veer MB, Behrendt H, Hahlen K, Sizoo W, Abels J: Characterization of the blast cells in acute leukemia with transloca-tion (4;11): Report of eight additional cases and of one case with a variant transloca-tion. Leukemia 1987;1:24–31.

13 Kaneko Y, Maseki N, Takasaki N, Sakurai M, Hayashi Y, Nakazawa S, Mori T, Saku-rai M, Takeda T, Shikano T, Hiyoshi Y: Clinical and hematologic characteristics in acute leukemia with 11q23 translocations. Blood 1986;67:484–491.

14 Katz F, Malcolm S, Gibbons B, Tilly R, Lam G, Robertson ME, Czepulkowski B, Chessels B: Cellular and molecular studies on infant null acute lymphoblastic leuke-mia. Blood 1988;71:1438–1447.

15 Krivit W, Good RA: Simultaneous occurrence of mongolism and leukemia. Am J Dis Child 1975;94:289–293.

16 Larson RA, Kondo K, Vardiman JW, Butler AE, Golomb HM; Rowley JD: Evidence for a 15;17 translocation in every patient with acute promyelocytic leukemia. Am J Med 1984;76:827–841.

17 Lewis DS, Thomspon M, Hudson E, Liberman MM, Samson D: Down's syndrome and acute megakaryoblastic leukemia: Case report and review of the literature. Acta Haemat 1983;70:236–242.

18   Miller RW: Persons with exceptionally high risk of leukemia. Cancer Res 1967;27:2420–2423.

19   Nagao T, Lampkin BC, Hug G: A neonate with Down's syndrome and transient abnormal myelopoiesis: serial blood and bone marrow studies. Blood 1970;36:443–447.

20   Roels F, Wisse E, De Brest B, von den Meulen J: Cytochemical discrimination between catalases and peroxidases using diaminobenzidine. Histochem 1975;41:281–311.

21   Shibata A, Bennett JM, Castoldi GL, Catovsky D, Flandirin G, Jaffe ES, Katayama I, Nanba K, Schmalzl F, Yam LT: Recommended methods for cytochemical procedures in haematology. Clin Lab Haematol 1985;7:55–74.

22   Stiller CA, Kinnier Wilson LM: Down's syndrome and leukemia. Lancet 1981;66:1343.

23   Tomonaga M, Yoshida Y, Tagawa M, Jinnai I, Kuriyama K, Amenomori T, Yoshioka A, Matsuo T, Nonaka H, Ichimaru M: Cytochemistry of acute promyelocytic leukemia (M3): Leukemic promyelocytes exhibit heterogeneous patterns in cellular differentiation. Blood 1985;66:350–357.

24   Vermaelen K, Barbieri D, Michaux J, Tricot G, Casteels-Van Daele M, Noens L, Van Hove W, Drochmans A, Louwagie A, Van Den Berghe H: Anomalies of the long arm of chromosome 11 in human myelo- and lymphoproliferative disorders. I. Acute nonlymphocytic leukemia. Cancer Genet Cytogenet 1983;8:105–116.

Dr. Angelo Cantù-Rajnoldi, Clinica del Lavoro,
Lab. Ematologia, I.C.P., Via San Barnaba, 8, I-20122 Milano (Italy)

Contrib Oncol. Basel, Karger, 1990, vol 41, pp 101–117.

Risk Factors in Neuroblastoma of Infants

F. Berthold[a], *D. Harms*[b], *F. Lampert*[c], *D. Niethammer*[d], *J. Zieschang*[a]

[a] Children's Hospital, University of Cologne
[b] Institute of Pathology, University of Kiel
[c] Children's Hospital, University of Gießen
[d] Children's Hospital, University of Tübingen, FRG

Zusammenfassung

Bei 258 Säuglingen mit Neuroblastom wurden prognostische Faktoren mittels univariater und multivariater Regressionsmodelle nach Cox untersucht und verglichen mit Patienten, die bei Diagnose älter als 1 Jahr waren. Im Säuglingsalter war die Zahl niederer Ausbreitungsstadien höher als bei älteren Kindern (Stadium I 19 %, II 15,5 %, III 26,0 %, IV 12,4 %, IV S 27,1 %). Außerdem kam ein differenziertes histologisches Bild (Hughes I⁰) so gut wie nicht vor. Alter per se (Säuglinge gegenüber Kindern über 1 Jahr) war ein wichtiger Risikofaktor. Wurden die Daten allerdings auf einer stadienbezogenen Basis analysiert, war die Bedeutung des Alters zu vernachlässigen. Bei Säuglingen mit lokalisiertem Neuroblastom (Stadium I bis III) waren hohe Ferritinwerte bei Diagnose und männliches Geschlecht ungünstige Risikofaktoren und erlaubten die Klassifizierung der Patienten in 3 Risikogruppen. Die ereignisfreien Überlebensraten für die 3 Gruppen waren 96 %, 67 % und 45 %. Bei Säuglingen mit Neuroblastom des Stadium IV S hatten der Allgemeinzustand bei Diagnose und die Resezierbarkeit des Primärtumors signifikanten Einfluß auf das ereignisfreie Überleben. Bedrohlich kranke Kinder, bei denen auch der Primärtumor nicht komplett entfernbar war, hatten eine ereignisfreie Überlebensrate von 0 %. Patienten mit besserem Allgemeinzustand bei Diagnose, jedoch inkompletter Entfernung des Primärtumors hatten eine ereignisfreie Überlebensrate von 77 % und Patienten mit vollständiger Entfernung des Primärtumors 100 %. Für Säuglinge mit Stadium IV waren hohe LDH bei Diagnose und Nichterreichen einer kompletten Remission ungünstige Faktoren. Die neuen Definitionen von Risikogruppen für Säuglinge mit Neuroblastom könnten von therapeutischer Relevanz sein.

Introduction

Neuroblastoma may be considered as *the* model neoplasm of infancy, not only for being the most frequent solid tumor during the first year of life

[1], but also because of the histology resembling to the corresponding embryonic tissues and the ability for maturation and regression [2]. Since the survival rate of the group of infants is much better compared to older children with neuroblastoma, age per se is taken as an independent prognostic factor by many authors [3 – 7]. The present study challenges this opinion on the basis of a close association between age and stage [8]. The retrospective analysis of data from 258 infants with neuroblastoma enabled us to identify risk factors in this age group and to define risk groups which allow to predict with some accuracy the outcome of the disease in these patients.

Patients and Methods

258 consecutive patients with age less than 365 days at diagnosis were analyzed retrospectively. They entered the GPO trials NB 79, NB 82 and NB 85 in cooperation with 77 Children Hospitals. The SAS statistical package and BMDP2L were used on a IBM Personal System/2 Model 60. For univariate risk factor analysis we used the Kaplan-Meier life table method comparing the curves by logrank and Wilcoxon tests (6.45 and 4.20). The following factors were investigated on a stage related basis: sex (male/female), age at diagnosis (0 – 11 months), general condition (normal activity, slightly reduced activity, reduced activity, distinctly reduced activity, critically ill), urinary catecholamine metabolites (normal/abnormal for age), serum LDH (normal/abnormal), serum ferritin (normal/abnormal), localization of the primary tumor (neck/thoracic/abdominal non-adrenal/adrenal/other/unknown), localization of metastases (bone marrow/bone/lymph nodes/liver/skin/central nervous system/other), number of metastatic sites, histological grade (Hughes' grades 1, 2, 3), utilization of therapeutic modalities (surgery/radiotherapy/chemotherapy), resectability of the primary tumor by inital or delayed surgery (biopsy/subtotal/total), achievement of remission (complete remission (CR)/partial remission (PR)/no remission (NR) including no change and progression). Univariatly identified risk factors were tested for possible correlation by the Mantel-Haenszel's chi-square test for contingency tables. If two or more factors were found to be correlated, the factor with the highest logrank p-value was chosen for further evaluation. For multivariate analysis the stepwise regression model was applied using the maximum partial likelihood ratio method presuming that the EFS rates were loglinear functions of the factors (Cox proportional hazards regression model).

The Cox regression model was applied to event free survival (EFS) data of the patients. EFS appeared to us more appropriate than survival (S), since in localized disease (stage I – III) and stage IV S neuroblastoma recurrences more often occur than death, while (with very few exceptions) death was preceded by reccurences. All patients had an observation time of more than 350 days. For multivariate analysis patients with missing values in one of the investigated variables had to be omitted. This resulted in a reduction of the patient population from 258 to 159 (stage I – III: from 156 to 72, stage IV S from 70 to 59, stage IV from 32 to 28).

Results

Influence of Age on the Distribution of Stages, Primary Sites, Tumor Markers and Grades

The stage distribution shows remarkable differences between infants with neuroblastoma and patients over one year of age (table 1). While in children over one year the number of patients increases with the stage, in infancy the number of stage I and II patients in considerably higher and metastatic disease in less frequent and mainly restricted to the special stage IV S type.

Infants of all stages experienced a survival rate of 84 % compared to 30 % for children over one year. A similar result is obtained for the event free survival rate (fig. 1). However, this comparison neglects the differences of the stage distribution between the age groups and of other risk factors. Figure 2 shows the Kaplan-Meier plots for stage III patients, which have been selected according to risk factors known to be important in older children [9]. These two curves run much closer although still different (logrank, Wilcoxon tests). For stage IV patients the EFS curves were not anymore statistically different. Risk adjusted overall survival curves were also not statistically different. Risk adjusted overall survival curves were also not statistically different for stage III and IV patients. As shown later with the Cox regression analysis age per se never proved to be an important risk factor.

No differences between infants and children over one year were observed among the distribution of primary sites. Similarly, the incidences of abnormal tumor marker levels including urinary catecholamine metabolites, lactic dehydrogenase, ferritin and neuron specific enolase were stage

Table 1. Stage distribution in infants with neuroblastoma compared to children over one year of age

Evans' stage	Infants (n = 258) %	Children > 1 year (n = 480) %
I	19.0	4.8
II	15.5	5.6
III	26.0	27.3
IV	12.4	62.1
IV S	27.1	0.2
	100.0	100.0

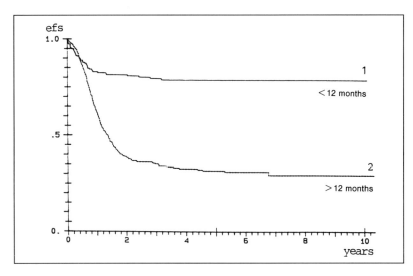

Fig. 1. Event free survival (EFS) in children with neuroblastoma of all stages without regard to different stage distribution (n = 738) NB 79/82/85. 11/89. 1. Infants < 12 months (n = 258; 49 events; EFS: 0.79 ± 0.03). 2. Children > 12 months (n = 480; 278 events; EFS: 0.29 ± 0.03).

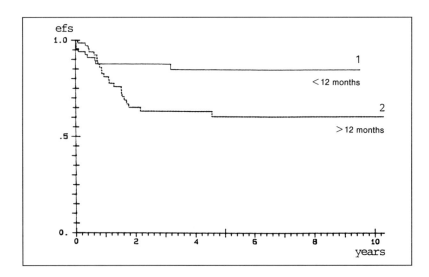

Fig. 2. Event free survival (EFS) in children with neuroblastoma stage III by age. The groups were risk factor adjusted (resectability, localization, ferritin) (n = 134) NB 78/82/85. 11/89. 1. Infants < 12 months (n = 67; 9 events; EFS: 0.84 ± 0.05). 2. Children > 12 months (n = 67; 23 events; EFS: 0.60 ± 0.06).

dependent as in older children. Table 2 summarizes the histologic patterns in 183 infants with untreated neuroblastoma using the modified Hughes classification [10, 11]. Grade 3 represents undifferentiated histology, grade 2 has signs of partial and grad 1 signs of complete differentiation at least in a few cells. In infancy the most differentiated type was present only in a negligible minority of cases (3 %) compared to 18 % in older patients. This may suggest a dependence of the maturation process from the age of life.

Influence of Stage on the Survival Rates

As in older children the event free survival of infants with stage IV was inferior compared to patients with localized (stages I, II, III) and stage IV S disease (logrank IV vs. I – III: 37.12 and IV vs. IV S: 6.39). The EFS prognosis for localized neuroblastoma was superior compared to IV S disease (logrank 8.10) (fig. 3). Infants qualified for stage IV (n = 32) mostly by bone metastasis (69 %), distant lymph node involvement (28 %), testicular tumor (12 %), CNS metastasis (9 %) and lung involvement (3 %). Unusual metastatic sites were predominant in the small group of infants in first half year of life and may represent a special subtype (CNS: 2 of 3 cases, testes: 2 of 4 cases). The survival rate of all infants was 84 % with no deaths later than 6 years after diagnosis (stage I – III 95 %, stage IV S 76 %, stage IV 48 %).

Stage Related Prognostic Factors

The estimation of prognostic factors was performed on a stage related basis, because stage is easily to define in an individual patient and because

Table 2. Incidence of histologic grades by stage in 183 infants with untreated neuroblastoma (all values in %)

Grade	Stage					
	I (n=39)	II (n=29)	III (n=49)	IV (n=21)	IV-S (n=45)	All (n=183)
1	5	10	–	–	–	3
2	48	45	53	24	38	44
3	46	45	47	76	62	54
Total	99	100	100	100	100	101
Anaplasia	3	3	2	10	2	3

of its overwhelming impact for prognosis. Three diagnostically clear-cut groups were defined, infants with localized neuroblastoma (Evans' stage I-III), infants with metastatic neuroblastoma (Evans' stage IV) and infants with stage IV S neuroblastoma (small primary, metastases restricted to liver, skin, bone marrow).

Localized disease: Age, general condition, primary site, catecholamine metabolites, lactic dehydrogenase, therapeutic modalities (chemotherapy versus radiotherapy versus chemo- and radiotherapy), resectability of the primary, histologic grading were not found to correlate with event free survival. Abnormal ferritin (fig. 4) and male sex (fig. 5) were associated with lower event free survival rates (table 3). No interrelationship between the two variables was found. These factors were selected for multivariate analysis and performed in the 72 patients for whom all data were available. Table 4 shows again the major impact of ferritin and minor importance of sex. These results permitted a classification of patients into 4 groups: group 1 ferritin normal, female; group 2 ferritin normal, male, group 3 ferritin abnormal, female; group 4 ferritin abnormal, male. Because of the identical curves of group 1 and 2 these patients were grouped together. The EFS curves of the resulting three risk groups are shown in figure 6.

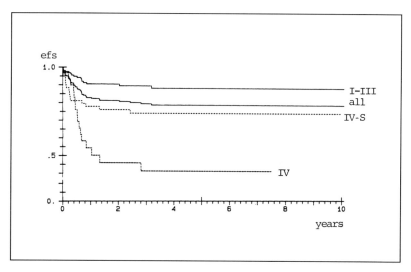

Fig. 3. Event free survival (EFS) in infants with neuroblastoma by stage (n = 258) NB 79/82/85. 11/89. I. Stage I-III (n = 156; 16 events; EFS: 0.88 ± 0.03). IV S. Stage IV S (n = 70; 17 events; EFS: 0.74 ± 0.05). IV. Stage IV (n = 32; 16 events; EFS: 0.41 ± 0.10). All stages (n = 258; 49 events; EFS: 0.79 ± 0.03).

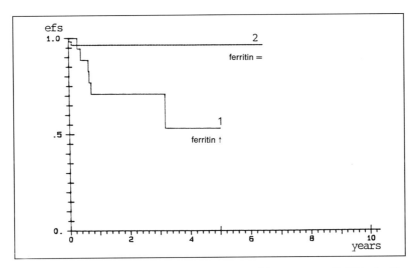

Fig. 4. Event free survival (EFS) in infants with neuroblastoma stages I – III by ferritin (n = 72) NB 79/82/85. 11/89. 1. Abnormal ferritin (n = 18; 6 events; EFS: 0.53 ± 0.17). 2. Normal ferritin (n = 54; 2 events; EFS: 0.96 ± 0.03).

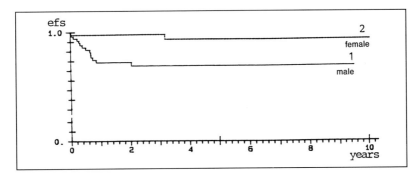

Fig. 5. Event free survival (EFS) in infants with neuroblastoma stages I – III by sex. NB 79/82/85. 11/89. 1. Male (n = 89; 14 events; EFS: 0.82± 0.04). 2. Female (n = 67; 2 events; EFS: 0.97 ± 0.03).

Table 3. Univariately identified risk factors for neuroblastoma stages I-III in infants

Risk factor	Definition of the risk factor	Logrank test *
Ferritin	abnormal (vs. normal)	11.82
Sex	male (vs. female)	7.27

* significance ≥ 3.84 ($\alpha = 0.05$)

Stage IV S disease: The event free survival in infants with stage IV S neuroblastoma was not influenced by age, sex, primary site, catecholamine metabolites, lactic dehydrogenase, ferritin, therapeutic modalities, histologic grading, metastatic site, number of metastatic sites and time of surgery (primary versus delayed).

The general condition of the infants as judged by the local physician was important for event free survival. 'Critically ill' patients had only a 15 % EFS chance compared to infants in a status of 'distinctly reduced', 'reduced', 'slightly reduced' or 'normal activity' at diagnosis with a 84 % EFS rate (fig. 7). A similar discrimination of two groups was obtained using the criteria 'complete remission achieved' (EFS: 0.91 ± 0.04, n = 50 (4 events) and

Table 4. Multivariately identified risk factors in infants with neuroblastoma stages I-III

Risk factor	ß	p	e^{β}
Ferritin (abnormal)	2.452	0.002	11.6120
Sex (male)	1.143	0.084	3.1381

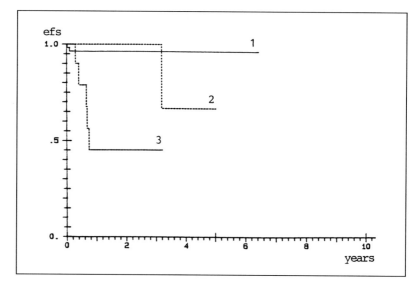

Fig. 6. Neuroblastoma stage I–III in infants. Event free survival (EFS) by risk groups (n = 72) NB 79/82/85. 11/89. 1. Group 1: ferritin normal, male or female (n = 54; 2 events; EFS: 0.96 ± 0.03), 2. Group 2: ferritin abnormal, female (n = 8; 1 event; EFS: 0.67 ± 0.27). 3. Group 3: ferritin abnormal, male (n = 10; 5 events; EFS: 0.45 ± 0.17).

'complete remission not achieved' (EFS 0.29 ± 0.10, n = 20 (13 events)). Furthermore the resectability of the primary tumor either be initial or by delayed surgery was important for the outcome (fig. 8, table 5). Using the Mantel-Haenszel's chisquare test an interrelationship between the factors 'general condition' and 'achieved complete remission' could be demons-trated (p = 0.002). This reduces the prognostic factors in stage IV S neuro-blastoma to general condition and resectability (table 6). Again, three risk groups were defined: group 1 (complete removal of the primary, any gen-eral condition) with 95 % EFS, group 2 (incomplete surgery, general condi-tion better than critically ill) with 77 % EFS and group 3 (incomplete surg-ery, critically ill) with 0 % EFS (fig. 9).

Stage IV disease: Sex, primary site, metastatic site, number of metas-tatic sites, histological grade, and resectability could be ruled out as prog-nostic factors by univariate analysis. Figure 10 shows the beneficial impact of an achieved complete remission in these infants and figure 11 the favor-able meaning of normal lactic dehydrogenase (LDH) levels at diagnosis. Other risk factors were abnormal ferritin, presence of liver metastasis, age less than 6 months and poor or moderate general condition (table 7). An interrelationship was found between LDH and ferritin (p = 0.020), between

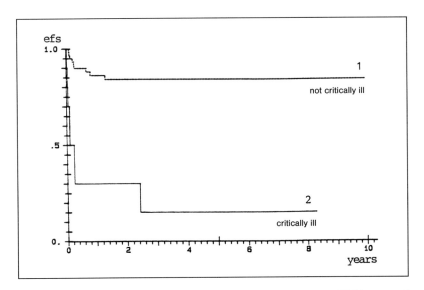

Fig. 7. Event free survival (EFS) in infants with neuroblastoma stage IV S by general condition at diagnosis (n = 70) NB 79/82/85. 11/89. 1. Better than critically ill (n = 60; 9 events; EFS: 0.84 ± 0.05). 2. Critically ill (n = 10; 8 events; EFS: 0.15 ± 0.13).

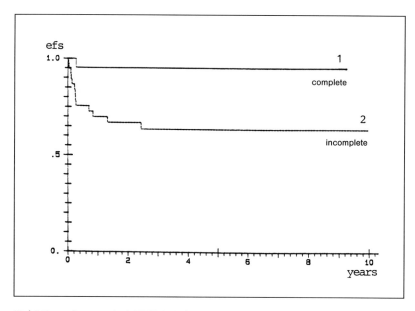

Fig. 8. Event free survival (EFS) in infants with neuroblastoma stage IV S by resectability of primary or delayed surgery (n = 59) NB 79/82/85. 11/89. 1. Total removal (n = 21; 1 event; EFS: 0.95 ± 0.05). 2. Subtotal removal, biopsy (n = 38; 13 events; EFS: 0.64 ± 0.08).

Table 5. Univariately identified risk factors for neuroblastoma stage IV S in infants

Risk factor	Definition of the risk factor	Logrank test *
General condition	critically ill (vs. better)	34.78
Resectability	total (vs. non-total)	6.44
Achieved CR	CR (vs. non-CR)	46.97

* significance ≥ 3.84 ($\alpha = 0.05$)

Table 6. Multivariately identified risk foctors in infants with neuroblastoma stage IV S

Risk factor	ß	p	$e^{ß}$
General condition	2.30	0.0002	9.9865
Resectability	2.08	0.0081	7.9655

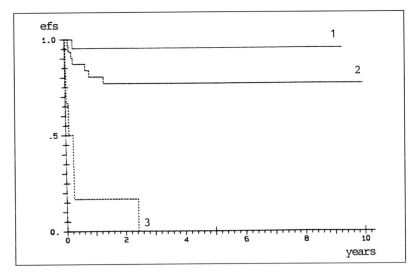

Fig. 9. Neuroblastoma stage IV S in infants. Event free survival (EFS) by risk groups (n = 59) NB 79/82/85. 11/89. 1. Complete removal, (n = 20; 1 event; EFS: 0.95 ± 0.05). 2. Subtotal removal or biopsy, general condition better than critically ill (n = 32; 7 events; EFS: 0.77 ± 0.08). 3. Subtotal removal or biopsy, critically ill (n = 6; 6 events; EFS: 0).

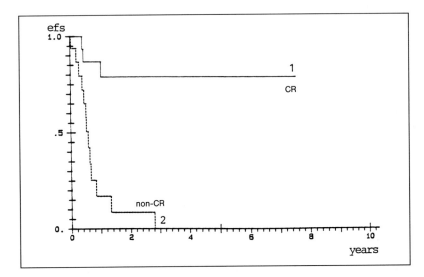

Fig. 10. Event free survival (EFS) in infants with neuroblastoma stage IV by achieved remission status (n =32) NB 79/82(85. 11/89. 1. Complete remission (n = 15; 3 events; EFS: 0.79 ± 0.11). 2. No complete remission (n = 17; 13 events; EFS: 0).

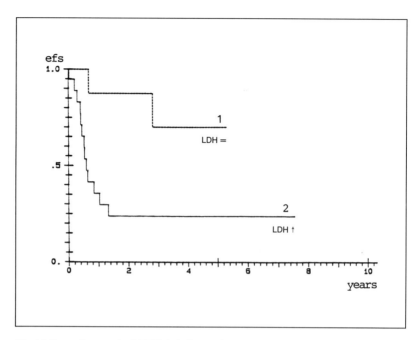

Fig. 11. Event free survival (EFS) in infants with neuroblastoma stage IV by LDH (n = 28) NB 79/82/85. 11/89. 1. Normal LDH (n = 8; 2 events; EFS: 0.70 ± 0.18). 2. Abnormal LDH (n = 20; 13 events; EFS: 0.24 ± 0.10).

Table 7. Univariately identified risk factors for neuroblastoma stage IV in infants

Risk factor	Definition of the risk factor	Logrank test *
Achieved CR	CR (vs. non-CR)	17.72
LDH	elevated (vs. normal)	5.54
Ferritin	elevated (vs. normal)	4.24
Liver metastasis	present (vs. absent)	3.97
Age	0–6 months (vs. 7–11 months)	5.73
General condition	poor vs moderate vs good +	6.25 **

* significance ≥ 3.84 ($\alpha = 0.05$)

** significance ≥ 5.99 ($\alpha = 0.05$)

+ poor: critically ill or distinctly reduced activity

  moderate: reduced or slightly reduced activity

  good: normal activity

age and liver metastasis (p = 0.025) and between general condition and liver metastasis (p = 0.031). The variables selected for multivariate analysis were remission status, LDH, age and general condition. The factors remission status and LDH sufficiently explained EFS data and further improvement was not achieved by inclusion of the other variables (table 8). The results permitted the classification of the patients into 4 risk groups (fig. 12): group 1 (CR and normal LDH) 100 % EFS, group 2 (CR, abnormal LDH) 57 %,

Table 8. Multivariately identified risk factors in infants with neuroblastoma stage IV

	ß	p	e$^\beta$
Remission (non-CR)	2.17	0.001	8.7626
LDH (abnormal)	1.45	0.033	4.2593

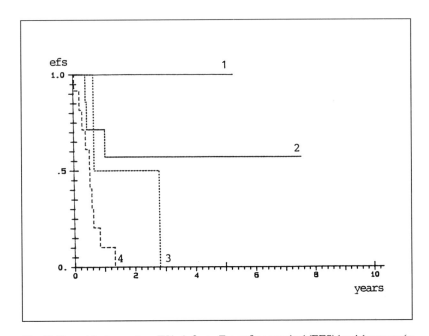

Fig. 12. Neuroblastoma stage IV in infants. Event free survival (EFS) by risk groups (n = 28) NB 79/82/85. 11/89. 1. Group 1: CR, normal LDH (n = 6; 0 events; EFS: 1.0). 2. Group 2: CR, abnormal LDH (n = 7; 3 events; EFS: 0.57 ± 0.19). 3. Group 3: PR or NR, normal LDH (n = 2; 2 events; EFS: O). 4. Group 4: PR or NR, abnormal LDH (n = 13; 10 events; EFS: 0).

group 3 (non-CR, normal LDH) EFS 0 % and group 4 (non-CR, abnormal LDH) EFS 0 %. Because of the small sample size, these categories should be regarded with some reservation.

Discussion

The accumulation of data from 258 infants out of a total of 738 patients made this first report on risk factor analysis for neuroblastoma in infancy possible. The patients were collected from the three consecutive trials NB 79, NB 82 and NB 85, where treatment of infants changed little over the time in stage I, II, III and IV S disease and showed no influence on the outcome in stage IV disease. The failing impact of risk factor 'therapy', which is considered extremely important in many other non-neuroblastoma trials, permitted us to use the compiled data of infants of all three trials.

Comparing the outcome of infants and children over one year of age on a stage related basis we found no major impact of the factor 'age'. This contrasts to other reports [3–7] where age was reported an important prognostic factor. However, these studies did not consider the change of the stage distribution with the age groups. The younger the patients the more low stage diseases were observed (table 1). For therapeutic reasons we chose 'stage' as the basic category for further risk factor analysis. No impact (stage I, II, IV, IV S univariately, all stages multivariately) or only moderate influence (stage III univariately, fig. 2) of the factor 'age' could be demonstrated comparing infants and children over 1 year of age.

Poor prognostic indicators in localized neuroblastoma were abnormal ferritin and male sex. They permitted the description of a good prognosis group with 96 % EFS (normal ferritin, male or female), of a intermediate group (abnormal ferritin, female) with 67 % EFS and a poor prognosis group (abnormal ferritin, male) with 45 % EFS. In older children ferritin has been reported as a prognostic factor before by several authors [5, 12, 13] and could be confirmed in our series for infants. Ferritin was not helpful to differentiate between stage IV S and stage IV in infancy.

The identification of general condition as the most important prognostic factor in stage IV S neuroblastoma defines the small proportion of infants with stage IV S which need therapy and may lead to a more active therapeutic attitude right from diagnosis in critically ill patients. An immediate start of chemo- or radiotherapy at diagnosis in these patients may prevent fatal progression at least in some of them. Furthermore the importance of the complete primary removal for prognosis provides a reason for a modified therapeutic attitude towards more surgical aggressiveness. A prognostic impact of age and pattern of metastases could not be confirmed in our series using the identical criteria as published [14].

True stage IV neuroblastoma is a rare disease in infancy (ratio IV S:IV disease 2.2:1). The 32 patients were collected over 10 years. The small sample size requires cautious interpretation of the results. However, abnormal LDH levels and failure to achieve complete remission are well conceivable risk factors, which discriminated four groups between 0 % and 100 % EFS in our series.

In conclusion, the multivariate analysis permitted the identification of stage related risk factors, which were based on simple clinical evaluations and tests. Variables which were not available during the early 80s (e.g. N-myc, chromosome 1 abnormalities, neuron specific enolase) have not been included in the analysis, but may prove to be independent risk factors in the future.

Summary

Prognostic factors were evaluated in 258 infants with neuroblastoma using univariate and multivariate regression models according to Cox and compared to the results in children over one year of age. The infants group was characterized by a higher number of low stage patients (stage I 19 %, II 15.5 %, III 26.0 %, IV 12.4 %, IV S 27.1 %) and by the nearly complete absence of mature histologic pattern (Hughes grade 1). Age per se (infants vs. children over 1 year) was an important risk factor. However, on a stage related basis, the impact was negligible. In infants with localized neuroblastoma (stage I–III), abnormal ferritin values at diagnosis and male sex proved to be risk factors and permitted classification of the patients into three risk groups. The event free survival rates for the three groups were 96 %, 67 %, 45 %. In infants with stage IV S neuroblastoma the general condition at diagnosis and the resectability of the primary tumor had a significant impact on EFS. Critically ill patients without total removal of the primary had an EFS rate of 0 %, while better general condition with incomplete removal resulted in 77 % and total primary removal with any general condition in 100 % EFS. For infants with stage IV abnormal LDH and failure to achieve complete remission were bad prognostic factors. The new definitions of risk groups for infants with neuroblastoma may be of therapeutic relevance.

Acknowledgement

The following Pediatric Hospitals contributed to this work: Aachen, R. Mertens; Augsburg, A. Gnekow, E. Pongratz; Bad Mergentheim, K. Rager; Bayreuth, G.F. Wündisch; Berlin, G. Henze; Bielefeld, V. Schöck; Bietigheim-Bissingen, Busch; Bochum, C. Mietens; Bonn, U. Bode; Braunschweig, G. Mau; Bremen, H.-J. Spaar; Burgwedel, D. Franke; Celle, G. Jacobi; Coesfeld, E. Lang; Darmstadt, Frauenknecht; Datteln, W. Andler; Detmold, Niemeyer; Dortmund, Breu; Düren, Johannsen; Düsseldorf, U. Göbel; Duisburg, H. Haupt; Erlangen, J.D. Beck; Essen, W. Havers; Frankfurt, V. Gerein; Freiburg, J. Holldack; Gießen, F. Lampert; Göttingen, M. Lakomek; Hamburg, Blunck, K. Winkler; Hannover, V. Hofmann, H. Riehm; Heidelberg, R. Ludwig; Heilbronn, H. Cremer; Herdecke, C. Tautz; Herford, Eisenberg; Herne, J. Engert; Homburg/ Saar, N. Graf; Iserlohn, F.-J. Knust; Kaiserslautern, I. Krüger; Karlsruhe, G. Nessler; Kassel, M. Wright, H. Wehinger; Kiel, Tuebben, R. Schneppenheim; Koblenz, M. Rister; Köln, W. Sternschulte, F. Berthold; Konstanz, H.-U. Schwenk; Krefeld, B. Dohrn; Ludwigshafen, H. Karte; Lübeck, J. Otte; Mainz, P. Gutjahr; Mannheim, O. Sauer; Marburg, C. Eschenbach; München, S. Müller-Weihrich, R.J. Haas, C. Bender-Götze, B. Heydenreich; Münster, J. Ritter; Neunkirchen, Feldmann-Ulrich; Neuwied, P.-M. Herding; Nordhorn, W. Hüther; Nürnberg, A. Jobke, P. Knoch; Osnabrück, von Mühlendahl, H. Rickers; Regensburg, Regenbrecht; Reutlingen, Rau; Rosenheim, Peller; Saarbrücken, R. Geib-König; Sankt Augustin, G. Verheyen; Schwäbisch Hall, H. Geiger; Schweinfurt, H. Giesen; Siegen, F.-J. Göbel; Stuttgart, J. Treuner; Trier, W. Heiss, Rauh; Tübingen, D. Niethammer; Ulm, G. Gaedicke; Wilhelmshaven, Krohn; Würzburg, J. Kühl; Wuppertal, N. Kuhn.

References

1   Kaatsch P, Michaelis J: Epidemiological data on childhood malignancies in the first year of life, in Lampert F (ed): Cancer in the first year of life. Contr Oncol. Basel, Karger, 1990, vol 41, pp 1–7.
2   Berthold F: Overview: Biology of Neuroblastoma, in Pochedly C, Tebbi C (ed), Neuroblastoma: Tumor biology and Therapy (in press).
3   Coldman AJ, Fryer CJH, Elwood JM, Sonley MJ: Neuroblastoma: Influence of age at diagnosis, stage, tumor site, and sex on prognosis. Cancer 1980;46:1896–1901.
4   Sandstedt B, Jereb B, Eklund G: Prognostic factors in neuroblastomas. Acta Pathol Microbiol Immunol Scand 1983;91:365–371.
5   Evans ED, D'Angio GJ, Propert K, Anderson J, Hann H-WL: Prognostic factors in neuroblastoma. Cancer 1987;59:1853–1859.
6   Carlsen NLT: Why age has independent prognostic significance and neuroblastomas. Evidence for intra-uterine development, and implications for the treatment of the disease. Anticancer Res 1988;8:255–262.
7   Oppedal BR, Storm-Mathisen I, Lie SO, Brandtzaeg P: Prognostic factors in neuroblastoma: Clinical, histopathologic, and immunohistochemical features and DNA ploidy in relation to prognosis. Cancer 1988;62:772–780.
8   Berthold F, Hunneman DH, Käser H, Harms D, Bertram U, Erttmann R, Schilling FH, Treuner J, Zieschang J: Neuroblastoma screening: Arguments from retrospective analysis of three German neuroblastoma trials. AmJ Pediat Hematol Oncol 1990 (in press).

9 Sieverts H: Good prognosis neuroblastoma. Results and further strategy. Minutes of the 21st meeting of the ENSG in Brussels, June 16 and 17th, 1989.
10 Hughes M, Marsden HB, Palmer MK: Histologic patterns of neuroblastoma related to prognosis and clinical staging. Cancer 1974;34:1706–1711.
11 Harms D, Wilke H: Neuroblastom-Grading. Klin Pädiat 1979;191:228–233.
12 Hann HL, Levy HM, Evans AE: Serum ferritin as a guide to therapy in neuroblastoma. Cancer Res 1980;40:1411–1413.
13 Hann HL, Evans Ae, Siegel SE, Wong KY, Sather H, Dalton A, Hammond D, Seeger RC: Prognostic importance of serum ferritin in patients with stages III and IV neuroblastoma: The Childrens Cancer Study Group experience. Cancer Res 1985;45:2843–2848.
14 Stephenson SR, Cook BA, Mease AD, Ruymann FB: The prognostic significance of age and pattern of metastases in stage IV–S neuroblastoma. Cancer 1986;58:372–375.

Prof. Dr. Frank Berthold, Universitäts-Kinderklinik,
Joseph-Stelzmann-Str. 9, D-5000 Köln 41 (FRG)

Contrib Oncol. Basel, Karger, 1990, vol 41, pp 118–128.

Neuroblastoma Under One Year of Age[1]

Clinical Aspects and Management

B. De Bernardi[a], *M. T. Di Tullio*[b], *L. Cordero di Montezemolo*[c],
S. Bagnulo[d], *M. Carli*[e], *A. Donfrancesco*[p], *A. Mancini*[f], *A. Acquaviva*[g],
A. Arrighini[h], *G. Bernini*[i], *M. Baligan*[g], *P. E. Cornelli*[t], *L. Felici*[j],
D. Gallisai[k], *G. Izzi*[o], *A. Moreno*[q], *L. Musi*[u], *A. Russo*[l], *P. Tamaro*[r],
R. Targhetta[m], *A. Zingone*[n], *P. Corciulo*[a], *L. Boni*[a], *P. Bruzzi*[v],
for the Italian Cooperative Group on Neuroblastoma

[a] Istituto 'Giannina Gaslini', Genoa; [b] Department of Pediatrics, University of
Naples; [c] Department of Pediatrics, University of Turin; [d] Department of
Pediatrics, University of Bari; [e] Department of Pediatrics, University of Padua;
[f] Department of Pediatrics, University of Bologna; [g] Department of Pediatrics,
University of Siena; [h] Department of Pediatrics, University of Brescia;
[i] Department of Pediatrics, University of Florence; [j] Department of Pediatrics,
University of Ancona; [k] Department of Pediatrics, University of Sassari;
[l] Department of Pediatrics, University of Catania; [m] Department of Pediatrics,
University of Cagliari; [n] Department of Pediatrics, University of Palermo;
[o] Department of Pediatrics, University of Parma; [p] Ospedale 'Bambino Gesù',
Rome; [q] Ospedale Niguarda, Milan; [r] Ospedale Infantile, 'Burlo-Garofalo',
Trieste; [s] Ospedale Maggiore, Bologna; [t] Ospedale Civile, Bergamo; [u] Ospedale
Civile, Vicenza; [v] Istitute Scientifico par la Ricerca sul Cancro, Genoa, Italy

Zusammenfassung

Innerhalb der Italienischen Neuroblastom-Kooperativgruppe wurden 671 Patienten
in der Zeit von 1979 bis 1988 registriert, wovon 183 Säuglinge waren. Hinsichtlich Stadien-
einteilung und Überleben, so gehörten davon 28 Patienten zur Gruppe 1 (26 überlebend);
37 zur Gruppe 2 (37 überlebend); 45 zur Gruppe 3 (36 überlebend); 28 zur Gruppe 4 (20
überlebend); 45 zur Gruppe 5 (Stadium IV-S, 40 überlebend). Interessanterweise gab es in
dieser Gruppe hinsichtlich Überlebensrate keinen Unterschied, ob eine Chemotherapie
mit oder ohne Peptichemio durchgeführt wurde. Die Gesamtüberlebensrate betrug 82 %
für unter 1 Jahr alte Patienten im Vergleich zu nur 31 % bei über 1 Jahr alten Patienten,
Säuglinge im Alter von 0–6 Monaten hatten sogar eine Überlebensrate von 86 %.

[1] Supported in part by Grant 88.00019.44 of the Italian National Research Council,
Special Project 'Oncology'

Introduction

Prognosis of neuroblastoma is influenced by several factors [1]; only two of them, however, age and tumor extension at diagnosis, are considered independent variables and are taken into account in the design of all therapeutic protocols for this disease [2, 3].

Regarding age, it is assumed that younger children have a better outcome. Few large series of cases uniformly staged and treated with prospective protocols, however, have been able to verify this assumption [4-6].

In this report, we have analyzed the clinical characteristics and course of children aged less than one year with neuroblastoma, diagnosed in 21 Italian pediatric Institutions over a ten-year period.

Material and Methods

Patients

Between January 1, 1979, and December 31, 1988, 671 children with neuroblastoma were registered in one of the Study Protocols designed by the Italian Cooperative Group on Neuroblastoma, an affiliation of the Italian Association for Pediatric Hematology and Oncology (A.I.E.O.P.). Of these 671 children, 584 were actually treated with the protocol to which they had been assigned. 183 out of 584 (31 %), aged less than one year at time of registration, represent the object of this analysis (table 1).

Patients' Staging

For patients with no evidence of tumor dissemination, disease extension was defined by surgical and pathologic criteria, as previously reported [7]; accordingly, children operated radically were included in group 1; those with minimal postoperative residue, and/or regional lymph node infiltration, in group 2; those considered not amenable to ablative surgery as judged by clinical and instrumental evaluation, or operated with a macroscopic residue presumably greater than 2 ml, in group 3. Children with evidence of tumor dissemi-

Table 1. Neuroblastoma. A series of the Italian Cooperative Group

Period of study	1979–1988
Cases registered	671
Cases treated with Cooperative Protocols	584
Cases under one year at diagnosis	183 (31 %)

nation represented group 4, with the exception of those who had characteristics predisposing to spontaneous tumor regression, i. e., age at diagnosis less than 6 months associated with metastatic involvement of liver, and/or bone marrow, and/or skin, but not of bone (group 5).

Treatment

Children in group 1 had no adjuvant therapy. Children in group 2 diagnosed before 1985 received adjuvant chemotherapy for approximately one month, consisting of two cycles of Peptichemio [8] separated by a 2-week interval; in both cycles the drug was given at a dose of 1.2 mg/kg for 5 consecutive days. Children diagnosed after January 1, 1985, received no adjuvant chemotherapy. Children in group 3 and 4 were treated by 4 consecutive protocols (labelled AIEOP NB-79, NB-80, NB-82, NB-85, respectively) according to the time of diagnosis; Protocol NB-85 was administered only to children aged ≥ 6 months.

Children in group 5 diagnosed before 1985 received two cycles of Peptichemio with the modalities described for group 2; for children diagnosed thereafter, the individual investigators were left free to give some kind of adjuvant therapy with the recommendation to avoid it unless clear evidence of tumor progression or deterioration of clinical status were observed.

Results

The number of new cases of neuroblastoma for each year of the 10-year study (all 584 cases treated with the group Protocols) ranged from 33 in 1979 to 78 in 1985 (median, 58). The percentage of cases in one year ranged from 18 % in 1979 to 40 % in 1985 (fig. 1). The distribution of cases in each month of life for the infants ranged from 11 in the third month to 20 in the sixth and eigth month (fig. 2). The main clinical characteristics of the 183 children aged less than one year at diagnosis are summarized in table 2.

Sex: There was a slight prevalence for the male sex (M/F ratio, 1.23), which was present in all groups, except in group 3, where the M/F ratio was 0.5.

Site of the primary: The abdomen was the original site of the tumor in 136 cases (74 %), the mediastinum in 24 (13 %), the thoraco-abdominal area in 4 (2 %), the pelvis in 5 (3 %), the lateral neck in 9 (5 %), other sites in 5 (3 %).

Disease extension at presentation: There were 28 children (15 %) in group 1, 37 (20 %) in group 2 (14 of them had tumoral infiltration of regional nodes), 45 (24 %) in group 3 (18 were 6 months old or younger), 27 (15 %) in group 4 (7 were 6 months old or younger), 45 (25 %) in group 5 (all aged 6 months or less with 19 of them under 2 months).

There was a preponderance of cases without metastases at presentation (110 vs. 73); among the 73 children with metastases, those with characteristics predisposing to spontaneous regression largely prevailed (45 children in group 5 vs. 28 in group 4).

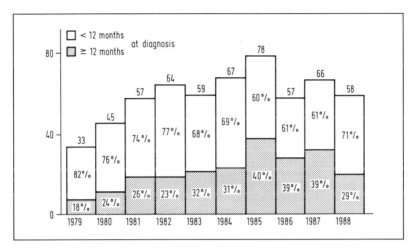

Fig. 1. Italian Cooperative Group on Neuroblastoma: Patient recruitment from 1979 to 1988 (584 cases).

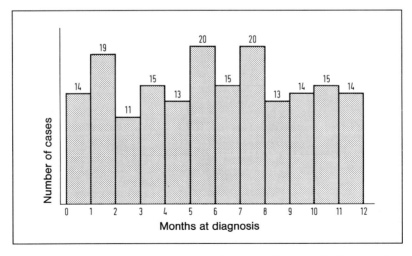

Fig. 2. Italian Cooperative Group on Neuroblastoma: 183 cases under 1 year at diagnosis. Registration for month of life.

Sites of metastases: In the 73 cases with metastases, the tumor spread was most frequent in the liver (52 cases, 71 %), followed by the bone marrow (32 cases, 44 %), the skin (19 cases, 26 %), the bone (13 cases, 18 %), the orbit (7 cases, 10 %), distant nodes (4 cases, 52 %). There were 7 cases with a miscellaneous of other sites involved.

Clinical course and survival: The actuarial overall survival (OS) for the entire series of 183 children with a median observation time of 35 months was 82 %, compared to an OS of 31 % in children aged $\geq$ 12 months as diagnosis (p < 0.0001) (fig. 3). The 107 children aged 6 months or less fared significantly better than the 76 aged between 6 and 12 months (OS: 86 % vs. 78 %, p=0.03) (fig. 4).

There was no difference in OS in relation to sex (85 % for male, 80 % for female sex; p=0.15). Regarding the site of primary, children with abdominal primary had a 82 % OS (88 % if the primary was in an adrenal, 76 % if the primary was in other abdominal locations; p=0.06), those with mediastinal primary at 100 %, those with other sites a 74 % (p=0.08).

Group 1: Of 28 such children, one died postoperatively, two (both aged 6 months at diagnosis) relapsed in bone marrow, and in bone + bone mar-

Table 2. 183 cases under one year at diagnosis. Clinical characteristics

Sex (M/F)	102/82
Primary	
abdomen	64
mediastinum	11
neck	5
other	4
pelvis	3
thoraco-abdominal	2
Disease Extension	(%)
localized	65 (35)
disseminated	73 (40)
inoperable	45 (25)
Metastatic Spread	
(73 cases)	
liver	52
bone marrow	32
skin	19
bone	13
orbit	7
other	7
distant nodes	4

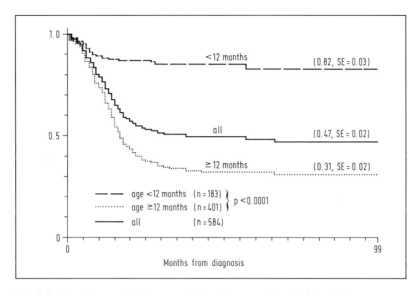

Fig. 3. Italian Cooperative Group on Neuroblastoma: Survival in relation to age at diagnosis (<12 vs ≥ 12 months).

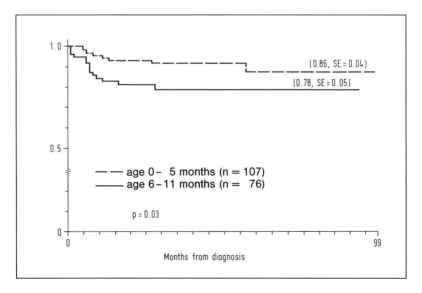

Fig. 4. Italian Cooperative Group on Neuroblastoma: Survival of cases diagnosed between 0–5 and 6–11 months of age.

row, at 17 and 52 months, respectively; of these two, the former is alive with disease at 16 months from relapse, the latter died 4 months after relapse due to an infectious complication.

26 of 28 children are alive and well at 1–99 months (median, 33 months) from diagnosis for an OS of 85 % (fig. 5).

Group 2: Of 37 such children (14 of whom with regional lymph node involvement), three (aged 5, 7, 11 months at diagnosis) relapsed locally at 4, 7, 3 months from diagnosis, respectively. Two out of the three had LN involvement at onset. All three were treated successfully and are presently alive and well at 18, 71 and 28 months from relapse, respectively.

OS is 100 % with a follow-up of 5–92 months (median, 40 months).

Group 3: Of 45 such children (18 aged <6 months), two died due to surgical complications; one died within two months from diagnosis due to Cisplatin toxicity.

Six children relapsed (1 out of the 18 aged < 6 months, 5 out of the 27 aged ≥6 months) at 3–5 months from diagnosis; in 5 of them relapse was local, in one it was local and in bone marrow. All 6 died of disease progression at 1–4 months from relapse. OS is 79 % with a follow-up of 0–89 months (median, 31 months). OS was better (p=0.05), for children aged <6 months (94 %), compared to 69 % of the 27 aged 6–11 months.

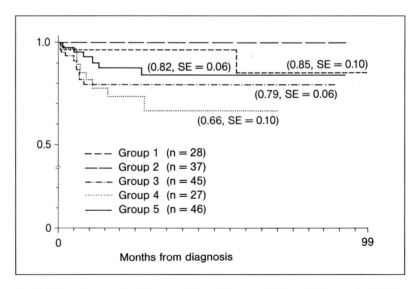

Fig. 5. Italian Cooperative Group on Neuroblastoma: NB under 1 year: Survival in relation to disease extension.

Group 4: Of 27 such children (7 aged < 6 months), one died shortly after diagnosis due to respiratory complications. Of the 26 evaluable, 7 relapsed (all >6 months) at 3-18 months (median, 5 months) from diagnosis. Relapses occurred locally in one case, in a disseminated form in 6 (also locally in 3 of them). Sites of distant relapses were bone marrow (one case), bone (3 cases), orbit (3 cases), distant nodes (2 cases). All these seven children died of disease at 1-13 months from relapse.

OS for the 27 children is 66% with a follow-up of 4-70 months (median, 23 months). OS was better, but not significantly, for the 7 children aged < 6 months (100%, vs. 58%; p=0.11) compared to the 20 aged ≥6 months.

Group 5: Of 46 such children, two, aged <1 month at diagnosis, died due to respiratory distress shortly after diagnosis; seven, aged 0, 0, 1, 1, 2, 5, and 5 months when first seen showed evidence of disease progression, or of relapse, at 4-19 months (median, 9 months) from diagnosis. Site of progression of relapse was local in one case, distant in 6 (three of them also local). Sites of progression or relapse were bone marrow in 3 cases, bone in 2, liver in 2.

Six of the 7 children who progressed or relapsed, including the three with local relapse, died at 1, 1, 3, 4, 8 and 8 months from time of progression or relapse. The remaining one is alive in CR at 5 years from relapse.

OS is 82% with a follow-up of 0-92 months (median, 30 months). Six/8 deaths occurred in the 19 children aged 0-1 month (OS, 65% vs 91% of children aged 2-5 months; p=0.04).

The 23 children registered before 1985 and treated with Peptichemio for 2 cycles have a 78% survival rate. The 23 registered thereafter, who received either no chemotherapy or 'free' chemotherapy on decision of the individual investigator, have an OS of 83% (p=0.81).

Discussion

Back in 1959, Gross et al. reported that children with neuroblastoma aged 0-11 months at diagnosis fare better compared with children aged 12-23, 24-35, 36-47 and ≥48 months (49%, vs. 24%, 14%, 9%, 6% respectively [9]. Since then, several authors confirmed that younger children have a more favourable clinical course and suggested that they probably deserve a less aggressive treatment to achieve permanent cure [1-6, 9, 10].

This report deals with a series of 183 consecutive children with neuroblastoma having less than one year of age at diagnosis. It differs from other reports on this issue, in that all children were staged according to a unique staging system [7] and were treated with prospective protocols.

The better outcome of children of this age group compared to older ones is confirmed by us: 82 % of our children survive with a median observation time of 35 months, against a 31 % survival of children aged $\geq$ one year.

In the 65 children operated radically or with minimal residue, there have been a total of 5 relapses, three of which were local; all local relapses occurred in cases operated with a minimal tumour residue (and 2/3 also had positive nodes) and could be rescued. It may be surprising that both disseminated relapses occurred in children who had been operated radically; this might mean that relapse was a consequence of tumor spread occurring before or during tumor ablation rather than of local tumor remnants.

Children with an inoperable primary were more suspectible to suffering from surgical and chemotherapy-related complications (3 deaths out of 45 cases). Six relapses occurred in 42 evaluable cases; despite the fact that 5/6 relapses were local, all 6 cases died, indicating a quite aggressive behaviour of the disease in recurrence. Relapses were more frequent in children aged more than 6 months; the difference, however, in survival compared to younger patients is not significant (70 % vs. 90 %).

Of the 27 children in group 4, one died of overwhelming disease before starting anticancer therapy, none died of surgical complications. Of the 7 relapses, only one was exclusively local; all occurred in children aged ≥ 6 months. The prevalence of relapses in bone and bone marrow replicates the pattern of relapses in older children. All seven relapses were followed by death from tumor progression. Also in group 4, survival is better for children younger than 6 months (100 %, vs. 58 %) without reaching the level of significance.

Of the 46 children in group 5 only two, aged less then one month, died of respiratory complications caused by an enormously enlarged liver. There were, however, 7 instances of clear disease progression of relapse, 5 of which disseminated (to bone and/or bone marrow), with 4 deaths. Six/7 instances of progression or relapse occurred in children aged less than 2 months at diagnosis; this confirms the opinion [11] that children of this group diagnosed in the first two months of life are at higher risk.

The OS of group 5 children (82 %) is similar to that reported by others [12–15]; it may be argued that, having included in this group only children under 6 months, a positive selection may have favored better results. Howeve-ver, only two of the 27 cases of our group 4 had characteristics of Evans' stage IV, and one of the two relapsed and died.

Summary

Within studies of the Italian Cooperative Group on Neuroblastoma, 671 patients were registered from 1979 to 1988, of whom 183 were infants. As to staging and outcome, there were 28 patients in group 1 (26 alive); 37 in group 2 (37 alive); 45 in group 3 (36 alive); 28 in group 4 (20 alive); 45 in group 5 (stage IV-S) (40 alive). Interestingly, there was no difference in survival in children of this group, whether chemotherapy with Peptichemio was given or not. Overall survival was 82 % for patients under one year of age as compared to only 31 % in patients over one year of age. Infants aged 0–6 months even had a survival of 86 %.

Acknowledgment

The authors are grateful to Ms. Roberta Boero and Ms. Anna Capurro for technical and secretarial assistance.

References

1   Evans AE, D'Angio GJ, Propert K, et al: Prognostic factors in neuroblastoma. Cancer 1987;59:1853–1859.
2   Jaffe N: Neuroblastoma: Review of the literature and examination of factors contri-buting to its enigmatic character. Cancer Treat Rev 1976;3:61–82.
3   Breslow N, McCann B: Statistical estimation of prognosis for children with neuro-blastoma. Cancer Res 1987;31:2098–2103.
4   Jereb B, Bretsky SS, Vogel R, et al: Age and prognosis in neuroblastoma. Am J Ped Hematol Oncol 1984;6:233–243.
5   Kinnier Wilson D, Draper GJ: Neuroblastoma. Its natural histoy and prognosis: A study of 487 cances. Br Med J 1974;3:301–307.
6   Berthold E, Brandeis WE, Lampert F: Neuroblastoma: Diagnostic advances and ther-apeutic results in 370 patients, in Riehm H (ed): Malignant neoplasma in childhood and adolescence. Monogr Paediat, Basel, Karger 1986, vol 18, pp 206–223.
7   De Bernardi B, Rogers D, Carli M, et al: Localized Neuroblastoma. Cancer 1987;60:1066–1072.
8   De Bernardi B, Comelli A, Cozzutto C, et al: Peptichemio in advanced Neuroblas-toma. Cancer Treat Rep 1978;62:811–817.
9   Gross RE, Farber S, Martin LW: Neuroblastoma sympatheticum. Pediatrics 1959;23: 1179–1191.

10   Carlsen NLT, Nielsen OH, Hertz H: Neuroblastoma. Acta Paediat Scand 1981;70: 61–66.

11   Wilson PG, Weitzman S, Coppes MJ, et al: Neuroblastoma Stage IV-S. Med Ped Oncol 1989;17:300.

12   Evans AE: Stage IV-S neuroblastoma. Med Ped Oncol 1979;6:85–91.

13   McWilliams NB, Hayes FA, Smith IE, et al: Stage IV-s Neuroblastoma: Chemotherapy vs. Observation. Proc Am Soc Clin Oncol 1986;5:211.

14   Stokes SH, Thomas PRM, Perez Ca, Vietti TJ: Stage IV-S neuroblastoma. Results with definitive therapy. Cancer 1984; 53:2083–2086.

15   Blatt J, Deutsch M, Wollmann MR: Results of therapy in Stage IV-S neuroblastoma with massive hepatomegaly. Int J Radiat Oncol Biol Phys 1987;13:1467–1471.

Dr. Bruno De Bernardi, Istituto 'Giannina Gaslini',
Via 5 Maggio 39, I-16147 Genova (Italy)

Contrib Oncol. Basel, Karger, 1990, vol 41, pp 129–135.

Cytogenetics of Neuroblastoma in Infancy

H. Christiansen[a], *W. Bielke*[a], *T. Cremer*[b], *F. Lampert*[a]

[a] Children's Hospital, University of Gießen
[b] Institute of Anthropology and Human Genetics, University of Heidelberg, FRG

Zusammenfassung

Bei 20 an Neuroblastom erkrankten Säuglingen ergab die Metaphasen-Zytogenetik eine Beschränkung der neuroblastom-spezifischen Chromosom 1p Deletion auf das klinische Stadium IV; dagegen war eine Multisomie von zytogenetisch normalen Chromosomen 1 charakteristisch für Neuroblastomtumore mit günstigem klinischen Verlauf. Diese Ergebnisse konnten durch eine neue Methode, die als Interphase-Zytogenetik bezeichnet wird, untermauert werden. Eine N-myc Onkogen-Amplifikation wurde ausschließlich im Stadium IV bei Säuglingen mit Neuroblastom gesehen.

Introduction

Cytogenetically, most prominent markers of neuroblastoma tumor cells are numerical and structural aberrations of chromosome 1 [3], including deletions of the short arm resulting in loss of genetic loci in defined chromosomal bands assigned as LOH (loss of heterozygosity) [5], the appearance of de-novo chromosomal material as DMs (double minute chromosomes) and HSRs (homogenously staining regions) [1], and different degrees of aneuploidy [6]. Molecular genetics revealed the proto-oncogene N-myc to be amplified in a subset of neuroblastoma tumors [2, 7]. The distribution within different clinical stages and prognostic meaning of these genetic markers will be discussed.

Classical metaphase cytogenetics is often hampered by poor quality of chromosome spreads of primary tumor material, low number of metaphases or no metaphases at all in about 70 % of tumors investigated with classical cytogenetic methods. To bypass these difficulties, we started to study chromosome number and structure independently from metaphases in interphase nuclei of neuroblastoma tumors. This is made possible by the use of chromosome specific repetitive DNA sequences in in-situ hybridizations performed on nuclei of primary tumors, yielding results in virtually all tumors investigated. First results will be represented.

Materials and Methods

Material

All patients investigated were registered within the neuroblastoma study of the German Society of Pediatric Oncology (GPO), which allowed the comparison of experimental with clinical data on the basis of standardized therapy protocols.

Standard Chromosome Analysis

Standard cytogenetic analyses were carried out on tumor and bone marrow samples cultured for 24 h. Karyotyping was performed after metaphase arrest by the addition of 0.01 μg/ml of Colcemid for 2 h, incubation with 0.075 M KCl, fixation by three changes of methanol/acetic acid (3:1 v/v), and a routine trypsin-Giemsa banding.

Interphase Cytogenetic Analysis

In-situ hybridization was carried out on cytogenetic preparations of methanol/acetic acid fixed nuclei. The probe used was a recombinant plasmid with a specific sequence from the satellite repeat families located near the centromere of chromosome 1 (pUC1.77) [4]. The probe was biotinated with bio-11-dUTP. For hybridization, 12.5 ng of the probe was used in a 50 μl hybridization mixture for each slide containing 65 % deionized formamide, 5 % dextransulfate, 2 $\times$ SSC, and carrier DNA (1 mg/ml sonicated salmon sperm DNA). The probe mixture and target were denatured together under a coverslip for 12 min at 73 °C in a moist chamber. Hybridization was performed for 16 h at 41 °C in an incubator. Slides were washed three times for 5 min each at 40 ° – 45 °C in 50 % formamide/2 $\times$ SSC, followed by three washes for 5 min with 0.1 $\times$ SSC at 55 ° – 60 °C.

The slides were subsequently treated with 1 $\times$ PBS/0.05 % Tween for 2 min, followed by 1 $\times$ PBS for 3 min. The biotinated probe was detected with peroxidase-conjugated streptavidin. The staining reaction (PBS/3,3-diaminobenzidine/H_2O_2) was performed for

10 min in the dark at room temperature. Slides were rinsed with tap-water for 10 min and air dried.

Results

Chromosome 1p aberrations were seen in none of the stage I, II and IVs tumors, however, in 1 of 2 stage III and 5 of 6 stage IV tumors. Numerical changes of chromosome 1 (trisomy til pentasomy) was encountered in all stage I, II and IVs tumors, whereas structural aberrations of the long arm of chromosome 1 was only seen in 1 of the 20 (= 5 %) neuroblastomas in infancy (a stage III tumor, table 1). Double minute chromosomes (DMs) or homogeneously staining regions (HSRs) were only detected in 4 out of 6 stage IV tumors correlating with the amplification of the N-myc proto-oncogene. In the absence of DMs or HSRs, a single copy of the proto-onco-gene N-myc per haploid genome was present.

In in-situ hybridizations with the chromosome 1 specific repetitive sequence pUC1.77 1000 nuclei were evaluated. The number of hybridiza-tion signals per nucleus were counted. Interphase cytogenetic analysis with pUC1.77 of a neuroblastoma stage II tumor with cytogenetic evidence of pentasomy of chromosome 1 showed more than 40 % of nuclei having five signals per nucleus (fig. 1). In a stage IV tumor, however, cytogenetically characterized by monosomy of chromosome 1, about 40 % of nuclei were positive for one signal (fig. 2). In this tumor, in addition to the great number of nuclei with a single signal per nucleus, about the same number showed two hybridization signals explainable by an additional tumor cell clone not detected by metaphase cytogenetics or by contamination of the nucleus preparation with non-tumor cells.

Table 1. Chromosome 1 aberrations and N-myc amplification in neuroblastoma in infancy

Stage	Total	1p−	1q+	+1	DMs/ HSRs	N–myc>1	1p⁻ and N–myc>1	+1 and N–myc=1
I	5	0	0	5	0	0	0	5
II	2	0	0	2	0	0	0	2
III	2	1	1	0	0	0	0	0
IV	6	5	0	0	4	4	4	0
IVs	5	0	0	5	0	0	0	5
Total	20	6	1	12	4	4	4	12

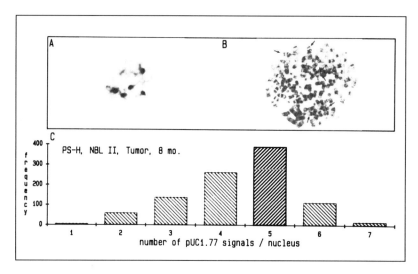

Fig. 1. Interphase cytogenetics of a stage II neuroblastoma (PS-H). A) Nucleus with 5 hybridization signals of pUC1.77. B) Metaphase of the same cell preparation with pentasomy of chromosome 1. C) Distribution of pUC1.77 signals per nucleus in 1000 nuclei evaluated.

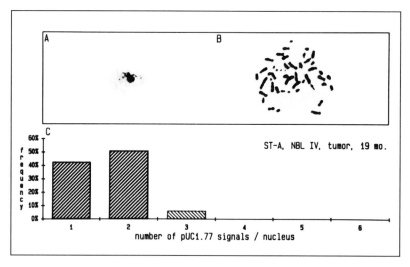

Fig. 2. Interphase cytogenetics of a stage IV neuroblastoma (ST-A). A) Nucleus with 1 hybridization signal of pUC1.77. B) Metaphases of the same cell preparation with monosomy of chromosome 1. C) Distribution of pUC1.77 signals per nucleus in 1000 nuclei evaluated.

Discussion

Cytogenetic analysis of neuroblastoma tumor cells is a very powerful tool in discriminating different prognostic entities. So far, structural aberrations of chromosome 1 have only been found in advanced neuroblastomas with a bad prognostic outcome, whereas chromosome 1 is cytogenetically normal in neuroblastomas with a favourable clinical course. Also, the chromosome number of the neuroblastoma tumor karyotype seems to influence prognosis. Especially chromosome numbers in the triploid range were found to correlate with a good prognostic outcome. In neuroblastoma of infancy, hyperploid tumor cells consistently revealed additional chromosomes 1, mostly resulting in trisomy of chromosome 1 (table 1). In conclusion, not only the absence of structural chromosome 1 aberrations but also the presence of numerical changes as trisomy of chromosome 1 is associated with a good prognosis. DMs and HSRs in neuroblastoma in infancy are restricted to stage IV tumors correlating with N-myc oncogene amplification. If DMs or HSRs are missing, the N-myc oncogene is always germline configurated. The molecular genetic analyses for N-myc amplification can readily be performed in all neuroblastoma tumors consecutively. However, classical metaphase cytogenetics is only successful in about 30 % of tumors investigated, but nevertheless contributes very important prognostic genetic markers as described above. To overcome these restrictions, we introduced interphase cytogenetic methods, which are able to delineate the configuration of single chromosomes on the level of intact nuclei independent from metaphases in all tumors studied. In neuroblastoma we will first concentrate on numerical changes of chromosome 1 by the use of a chromosome 1 specific repetitive sequence. With the help of this interphase approach, having in mind the metaphase results of numerical changes of chromosome 1 and its prognostic meaning, we want to classify neuroblastomas in two different entities. A majority of neuroblastoma tumor cell nuclei showing three or more hybridization signals per nucleus describes one subentity, a majority of nuclei with two or one hybridization signal per nucleus characterizes the other (table 1).

All tumors are then consecutively investigated for numerical changes of chromosome 1 by interphase cytogenetics and for N-myc oncogene amplification by molecular genetics.

The worst clinical outcome is assumed in tumors characterized by the combined presence of pUC1.77 signals per nucleus being two or one and N-myc amplification, whereas pUC1.77 signals per nucleus being three or more without N-myc amplification should confer the best prognostic outcome onto patients with neuroblastoma.

The elaboration of interphase cytogenetics of chromosome 1 by the combination of different chromosome 1 specific repetitive sequences localized in different defined chromosome bands will further allow the study of structural aberrations as the 1p deletion. This will lead to a more reliable subdivison of neuroblastoma in two different clinical entities with the help of genetic markers.

Summary

In 20 infants with neuroblastoma, metaphase cytogenetic analyses revealed the chromosome 1p deletion to be restricted to advanced clinical stages, whereas multisomy of cytogenetically inaberrant chromosomes 1 was characteristic for neuroblastoma with a favourable prognostic outcome. These results could be emphazised by a new method termed interphase cytogenetics. In infancy, N-myc oncogene amplification was seen only in stage IV tumors of neuroblastoma.

Acknowledgements

The excellent technical assistence of Miss Rosel Engel is appreciated. This study was supported by the Deutsche Forschungsgemeinschaft (La 185/8-1).

References

1   Biedler JL, Spengler BA: A novel chromosome abnormality in human neuroblastoma and antifolate-resistant Chinese hamster cell lines in culture. J Natl Cancer Inst 1976;57:683–695.

2   Brodeur GM, Seeger RC, Schwab M, Varmus HE, Bishop JM: Amplification of N-myc in untreated human neuroblastomas correlates with advanced disease stage. Science 1984;224:1121–1124.

3   Christiansen H, Lampert F: Tumour karyotype discriminates between good and bad prognostic outcome in neuroblastoma. Br J Cancer 1988;57:121–126.

4   Cooke HJ, Hindley J: Cloning of human satellite III DNA: different components are on different chromosomes. Nucl Acids Res 1979;6:3177–3197.

5   Fong CT, Dracopoli NC, White PS, Merrill PT, Griffith RC, Housman DE, Brodeur GM: Loss of heterozygosity for the short arm of chromosome 1 in human neuroblastomas: Correlation with N-myc amplification. Proc Natl Acad Sci USA 1989; 86:3753–3757.

6   Kaneko Y, Kanda N, Maseki N, Sakurai M, Tsuchida Y, Takeda T, Okabe I, Sakurai
     M: Different karyotypic patterns in early and advanced stage neuroblastomas. Cancer
     Res 1987;47:311–318.
7   Seeger RC, Brodeur GM, Sather H, Dalton A, Siegel SB, Wong KY, Hammond D:
     Association of multiple copies of the N-myc oncogene with rapid progression of neu-
     roblastomas. N Engl J Med 1985;313:1111–1116.

Dr. Holger Christiansen, Universitäts-Kinderpoliklinik,
Feulgenstraße 12, D-6300 Gießen (FRG)

Contrib Oncol. Basel, Karger, 1990, vol 41, pp 136–152.

Age-dependent Prognostic Significance of N-myc Copy Number in Neuroblastoma[1]

G. P. Tonini[a], *M. Badiali*[b], *A. Cavazzana*[d], *D. Di Martino*[a],
C. Dominici[c], *V. Fontana*[f], *A. Iolascon*[e], *E. Lanino*[a], *G. Basso*[d],
A. Pession[b], *G. Raschellá*[c], *P. Strigini*[f], *R. Sansone*[f], *B. De Bernardi*[a]

[a] Pediatric Oncology, Gaslini Children's Hospital, Genoa
[b] University of Bologna
[c] University of Rome
[d] University of Padua
[e] University of Naples
[f] Institute for Cancer Research, Genoa, Italy

Zusammenfassung

Zwischen Januar 1984 und Dezember 1988 wurden 107 Neuroblastom (Nb)-Frischtumoren (inklusive 53 Patienten weniger als 1 Jahre alt zur Zeit der Diagnose) auf N-myc Amplifikation (NMA) untersucht. Zusätzlich wurde NMA mit u. a. folgenden für die Prognose wichtigen biologischen und klinischen Variablen korreliert: Klinisches Stadium [1,2], histologisches Grading [3], urinäre Ausscheidung von Vanillinmandelsäure (VMA) und Homovanillinsäure (HVA); Serumspiegel von Ferritin (Fer), neuronspezifische Enolase (NSE) und Laktatdehydrogenasen (LHD); und Volumen (Vol) des primären Tumors. Diese Korrelationen wurden unter allen 107 Patienten und in der Säuglingsgruppe (Alter ≤ 1 Jahr) ausgewertet.

N-myc war amplifiziert in 7/53 < 1 Jahr (0/4 Stadium I, 0/8 Stadium II, 2/16 Stadium III, 3/13 Stadium IV, 2/12 Stadium IV-S) und in 12/54 Nb ≥ 1 Jahr (0/5 Stadium I, 0/5 Stadium II, 5/11 Stadium III, 7/32 Stadium IV, 0/1 Stadium IV-S). Die Gesamtverbreitung von NMA ist wesentlich niedriger als die von Seeger et al. in USA [4] und Tsuda et al. in Japan [5] beobachtet. Unter allen Probanden wurde NMA mit einer schlechteren Prognose in Verbindung gebracht.

Eine Analyse der gemeinsamen Verteilung von N-myc und Histologie [3] offenbarte keine signifikante Korrelation zwischen diesen beiden Variablen. Unter den analysierten Tumormarkern wurden niedrige VMA-Spiegel und hohe Spiegel von NSE und LDH mit NMA in älteren Kindern in Verbindung gebracht, in Säuglingen jedoch nicht.

Obwohl der Wert der NMA als prognostischer Indikator durch diese Studie bestätigt wurde, bedarf er einer Qualifikation. Die Bedeutung der NMA als Faktor der Tumorprogression muß weiter untersucht werden. Die Korrelationen mit anderen Malignitätsmar-

[1] Italian Neuroblastoma Research Program of the Italian Association of Pediatric Hematology/Oncology (A.I.E.O.P.)

kern mögen aufschlußreich sein. Die verschiedenen Muster dieser in Säuglingen und älteren Kindern gefundenen Markern könnten in der Lage sein, den prognostischen Wert von N-myc zu verfeinern und die Geschichte von Nb zu verstehen.

Introduction

Neuroblastoma is the most common neoplasm diagnosed at birth [6] as well as in children under one year of age; its incidence declines rapidly after the age of 2 years. This high incidence in infancy has suggested prezygotic or prenatal factors [8], either genetic [9] or environmental [10]. According to Knudson [8], malignant Nb cells carry two homologous mutations, the first occuring either pre or post-zygotically, the second being always post-zygotic. Timing of the first mutation defines true congenital versus non-congenital cases. Some early cases (stage IV–S), however, which may involve other locations besides the adrenal gland, might represent non-malignant hyperplastic nodules of primitive neuroblasts [11].

Two major molecular abnormalities have been detected in cancer cells of most advanced Nb cases [11 b]:

1. 1p32pter deletions [12, 12 b, 12 c], presumably involving the antioncogene mutation postulated by Knudson;

2. Amplification [4, 5, 13–16] and/or overexpression [17–20] of a cellular oncogene, dubbed N-myc, which is correlated with clinical aggressiveness and worse prognosis [4, 5, 13–20]. NMA has been rarely detected in non-advanced Nb [4, 5, 13–17, 21–24] as well as in infants [4, 5, 15–17, 21–23, 25] and its significance in such categories is still controversial [21, 22, 22 b].

We present a new series of cases of Nb and analyze the correlation between N-myc copy number and some bio-clinical variables and prognosis. Our data show peculiar differences at the molecular level between infants and elder ones.

Materials and Methods

Tumor samples were obtained from patients diagnosed to have Nb between 1978 and 1987. Clinical staging was performed according to Evans [1] and De Bernardi [2]. Some cases were evaluated after chemotherapy administration and during relapse. Histological classification was made according to Mäkinen [3].

DNA extraction, purification, digestion with endonuclease enzyme EcoRI, and Southern blotting were performed as previously described by Maniatis et al. [26], with minor modifications [27–29], and the samples were hybridized with [^{32}P]-labeled EcoRI-EcoRI insert derived by N-myc probe NB 19–20 (kindly provided by F. W. Alt, Columbia University, New York), and by Nb1 probe (kindly provided by J.M. Bishop, Los Angeles University, Los Angeles, CA). The value of NMA was calculated by comparison of Southern blot by densitometric analysis. DNA from SK-N-SH and IMR 32 human cell lines were used as negative and positive controls, respectively.

Statistical analysis of N-myc and other biological variables of clinical and prognostitc significance to evaluate correlations was performed according to Pearson [30]. In some analyses we grouped treated and untreated cases, because N-myc copy number seems to be substantially unchanged by chemotherapy [31, 32]. In the analysis of the correlations between NMA and other bio-clinical variables, amplification has been expressed as the log of N-myc copy number to allow analysis of the entire range of variation, taking into account the plausible biological mechanism of N-myc duplication [33–35].

Given the different methods used in urinary catecholamine evaluation, we transformed the observed values in multiples of standard deviation. Progression-free survival, defined as survival without progressive tumor growth, was used as the measure of outcome. Product-limit method was applied to estimate progression-free survival curves [36]. Differences between two curves were evaluated by means of Mantel-Cox and Breslow tests [37, 38].

Results

Correlation of N-myc copy number with age and stage. Tables 1 and 2 show the distribution of N-myc copy numbers by age and by clinical stage at onset [45]. NMA was present in 7/53 (13.2%) of patients less than 1 year old at diagnosis and in 12/54 (22.2%) in elder children, with no significant difference between the two groups.

Amplification was detectable in none of 6 cases in stage I, 0 out of 13 cases in stage II, 7 out of 27 (25.9%) in stage III, 10 out of 45 (22.2%) in stage

Table 1. Distribution of N-myc copies by age at diagnosis

N-myc copies	Age (years)		Total
	< 1	≥ 1	
< 3	46 (43 %)	42 (39.3 %)	88 (82.2 %)
≥ 3	7 (6.5 %)	12 (11.2 %)	19 (17.8 %)
Total	53 (49.5 %)	54 (50.5 %)	107 (100 %)

Chi-Square = 0.93511; P = 0.3335
Number of missing observations = 0

IV, and 2 out of 13 (15.4%) in stage IV–S. A comparison between the distribution of NMA within advanced (III and IV) and non-advanced stages (I, II and IV – S) shows a significant excess of amplified cases in the former group (P<0.05).

Table 3 shows the joint distribution of N-myc and Evans stages by age at onset (cut-off, 1 year). Among infants, N-myc amplification was present in 0/4 stage I, 0/8 stage II, 2/16 (12.5%) stage III, 3/13 (23%) stage IV, 2/12 (16.7%) stage IV – S, whereas in non-infants it was present in 0/5 stage I, 0/5 stage II, 5/11 (45.5%) stage III, 7/32 (21.9%) stage IV and 0/1 stage IV–S. Finally, table 4 compares the prevalence of NMA within advanced stages (III and IV) in Italian Nb cases versus U.S. [4] and Japanese cases [5]. Italian cases seem to be amplified less frequently than U.S. or Japanese counterparts (P<0.001).

Correlation between NMA and histologic grade. Table 5 presents the correlation between N-myc and histology (staged according to Mäkinen [3]). NMA was detectable in 9/33 (27.3%) grade I, 2/25 (8%) grade IIa, and 1/15 (6.7%) grade IIb. Comparing the prevalence of N-myc amplified cases in grade I versus grade IIa and IIb cumulated, a difference very close to the nominal level of significance was found (chi square=3.808; P=0.051 with one degree of freedom). No remarkable differences are detectable by age stratification (table 6).

Correlation between N-myc copy number and other bio-clinical variables of prognostic significance. Table 7 shows the correlations between N-myc copies and biochemical variables. In all but 12 cases, N-myc copy number was evaluated at onset. All the other variables were evaluated at onset: VMA, HVA, Fer, LDH, NSE, and volume of the primary tumor. N-myc is positively correlated with serum levels of LDH and NSE. This association is

Table 2. Distribution of N-myc copies by Evans' stage

N-myc copies	Stage					
	I	II	III	IV	IV–S	Total
<3	9 (8.4%)	13 (12.1%)	20 (18.7%)	35 (32.7%)	11 (10.3%)	88 (82.2%)
≥3			7 (6.5%)	10 (9.3%)	2 (1.9%)	19 (17.8%)
Total	9 (8.4%)	13 (12.1%)	27 (25.2%)	45 (42.1%)	13 (12.1%)	107 (100%)

Chi-Square = 6.64821, P = 0.1557
Number of missing observations = 0

Table 3a and b. Distribution of N-myc copies by Evans' stage and age at diagnosis. *a.* Age < 1 year.

N-myc copies	Stage					
	I	II	III	IV	IV-S	Total
< 3	4 (7.5 %)	8 (15.1 %)	14 (26.4 %)	10 (18.9 %)	10 (18.9 %)	46 (86.8 %)
≥ 3			2 (3.8 %)	3 (5.7 %)	2 (3.8 %)	7 (13.2 %)
Total	4 (7.5 %)	8 (15.1 %)	16 (30.2 %)	13 (24.5 %)	12 (22.6 %)	53 (100 %)

Chi-Square = 3.06297, P = 0.5

b. Age ≥ 1 year

N-myc copies	Stage					
	I	II	III	IV	IV-S	Total
< 3	5 (9.3 %)	5 (9.3 %)	6 (11.1 %)	25 (46.3 %)	1 (1.9 %)	42 (77.8 %)
≥ 3			5 (9.3 %)	7 (13.0 %)		12 (22.2 %)
Total	5 (9.3 %)	5 (9.3 %)	11 (20.4 %)	32 (59.3 %)	1 (1.9 %)	54 (100 %)

Chi-Square = 6.58015, P = 0.1598
Number of missing observation = 0

Table 4. Prevalence of N-myc copies within advanced stages (III and IV) in Italy, USA (4) and Japan (5)

N-myc copies	Country			
	Italy	USA	Japan	Total
< 3	55 (34.2 %)	28 (17.4 %)	13 (8.1 %)	96 (59.6 %)
≥ 3	17 (10.5 %)	32 (19.9 %)	16 (9.9 %)	65 (40.4 %)
Total	72 (44.7 %)	60 (37.3 %)	29 (18.0 %)	161 (100 %)

Chi-Square = 15.231; P = 0.0005

Table 5. Distribution of N-myc copies by Mäkinen histologic classification

N-myc copies	Grade			
	I	II a	II b	Total
< 3	24 (32.9 %)	23 (31.5 %)	14 (19.2 %)	61 (83.6 %)
≥ 3	9 (12.3 %)	2 (2.7 %)	1 (1.4 %)	12 (16.4 %)
Total	33 (45.2 %)	25 (34.2 %)	15 (20.5 %)	73 (100 %)

Chi-Square = 5.15872; P = 0.0758
Number of missing observations = 34

Table 6a and b. Distribution of N-myc copies by Mäkinen classification (grades II a & II b cumulated) and by age at diagnosis. *a.* Age < 1 year.

N-myc copies	Grade		
	I	II a + II b	Total
< 3	13 (32.5 %)	21 (42.5 %)	34 (85.0 %)
≥ 3	4 (10.0 %)	2 (5.0 %)	6 (15.0 %)
Total	17 (42.5 %)	23 (57.5 %)	40 (100 %)

Chi-Square = 0.72414; P = 0.3948

b. Age ≥ 1 year

N-myc copies	Grade		
	I	II a + II b	Total
< 3	11 (33.3 %)	16 (48.5 %)	27 (81.8 %)
≥ 3	5 (15.2 %)	2 (3.0 %)	6 (18.2 %)
Total	16 (48.5 %)	17 (51.5 %)	33 (100 %)

Chi-Square = 2.06419; P = 0.1508
Number of missing observations = 34

statistically significant (P<0.01 in both cases). Considering the whole group, no other variables are significantly correlated with the N-myc copy number. By contrast, stratifying the sample by age at diagnosis (cut-off, 1 year) (Tables 8–10), it is possible to note that:

1. Another variable (VMA) shows a significant negative correlation (–0.35, 53 evaluated cases) with NMA in patients ≥ 1 year at onset, with

Table 7. Correlations between N-myc copies and other bio-clinical variables (in brackets number of evaluated cases)

	VMA	HVA	LDH	NSE	Fer	Age	Vol	MYC
VMA	1.00							
HVA	0.36[a] (67)	1.00						
LDH	–0.11 (75)	0.06 (54)	1.00					
NSE	–0.18 (20)	–0.22 (20)	0.74[b] (20)	1.00				
Fer	–0.09 (67)	0.03 (49)	0.14 (68)	0.17 (17)	1.00			
Age	–0.10 (88)	0.02 (67)	0.02 (79)	0.27 (20)	0.25 (72)	1.00		
Vol	0.00 (38)	0.29 (32)	0.14 (33)	0.22 (17)	–0.10 (28)	0.17 (39)	1.00	
MYC	–0.15 (91)	–0.09 (68)	0.58[b] (80)	0.74[b] (20)	0.02 (73)	–0.06 (104)	0.29 (40)	1.00

VMA: Vanilliylmandelic acid, HVA: homovanillic acid, LDH: lactic dehydrogenase, NSE: neuron specific enolase, Fer: serum ferritin, Vol: Volume of primary tumor, MYC = Log_e (N-myc)

[a] $p < 0.05$
[b] $p < 0.01$

Table 8. Correlations between N-myc copies and other bio-clinical variables in patients <1 year at diagnosis (in brackets number of evaluated cases)

	VMA	HVA	LDH	NSE	Fer	Vol	MYC
VMA	1.00						
HVA	0.41 (25)	1.00					
LDH	–0.10 (27)	0.13 (19)	1.00				
NSE	–0.03 (8)	–0.15 (8)	0.60 (8)	1.00			
Fer	–0.16 (27)	0.18 (19)	0.31 (27)	–0.38 (7)	1.00		
Vol	0.31 (11)	0.28 (10)	0.45 (9)	0.31 (5)	–0.34 (9)	1.00	
MYC	–0.09 (35)	–0.13 (25)	0.01 (30)	–0.40 (8)	0.04 (29)	0.52 (12)	1.00

MYC = Log_e(N-myc)

For abbreviations see table 7.

little correlation in infants; the difference between the correlation coefficients of the two groups, however, is not statistically significant (Table 10).

2. The correlation between N-myc copy number versus NSE and LDH are -0.58 and 0.76 in non-infants, and -0.40 and 0.01 in infants, respectively. Such a difference is statistically significant in both cases (Table 10).

Correlation of N-myc amplification with prognosis. In 87 out of 98 samples collected at the onset, we analyzed the correlation between N-myc copy numbers and prognosis, expressed as PFS (fig. 1). The PFS rate in

Table 9. Analysis of the correlations between N-myc copies and other bio-clinical variables in patients ≥ 1 year at diagnosis (in brackets number of evaluated cases)

	VMA	HVA	LDH	NSE	Fer	Vol	MYC
VMA	1.00						
HVA	0.55[b] (41)	1.00					
LDH	−0.26 (47)	0.08 (35)	1.00				
NSE	−0.44 (12)	−0.37 (12)	0.69 (12)	1.00			
Fer	0.08 (39)	−0.15 (30)	0.09 (40)	0.08 (10)	1.00		
Vol	0.07 (26)	0.32 (22)	0.06 (24)	0.15 (12)	−0.15 (19)	1.00	
MYC	−0.35[a] (53)	−0.09 (42)	0.58[b] (50)	−0.76[a] (12)	−0.06 (43)	0.32 (27)	1.00

$MYC = Log_e(N\text{-myc})$

[a] $p < 0.05$
[b] $p < 0.01$

For abbreviations see table 7.

Table 10. Correlation coefficients of N-myc copy number versus bio-clinical variables by age group

Variables	<1 year	≥1 year	Test
VMA	−0.09 (35)	−0.35 (53)	−1.216
HVA	−0.13 (25)	−0.09 (42)	0.152
LDH	0.01 (30)	0.58 (50)	2.702[a]
NSE	−0.40 (8)	0.76 (12)	2.545[a]
Fer	0.04 (29)	−0.06 (43)	−0.397
Vol	0.52 (12)	0.32 (27)	−0.626

[a] $p < 0.01$

For abbreviations see table 7

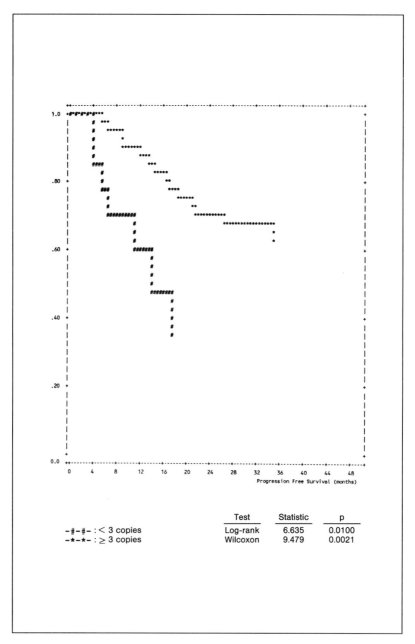

Fig. 1. Progression free survival estimated by Kaplan-Meier method (87 cases at onset).

patients with amplification of N-myc (equal to or more than 3 copies per haploid genome) is associated with a significantly worse prognosis compared to non-amplified cases (Wilcoxon test=9.479, P=0.0021; Log-rank test=6.635, P=0.010). A statistically significant worse prognosis in N-mycamplified cases was also present if the PFS analysis is restricted to advanced cases (stages III & IV) (Wilcoxon test=13.084; P=0.0003; Log-rank test=12.115; P=0.0005).

PFS of advanced stages has been also analyzed after stratification by age at onset (cut-off, 1 year). A significant association between NMA and shorter PFS has been found in both age groups, although definitely stronger in infant cases (fig. 2, 3).

Finally, PFS of advanced cases has been stratified by the N-myc copy number (cut-off, 3 copies). Whereas, within non-amplified cases, infants show a significantly better prognosis than non-infants (fig. 4), no such difference is detectable in amplified cases (fig. 5).

Discussion

Nb is presently considered a heterogeneous disease displaying a great clinical variability. Depending on the extent of the disease, patients can be placed into at least five groups with different prognosis. However, additio-

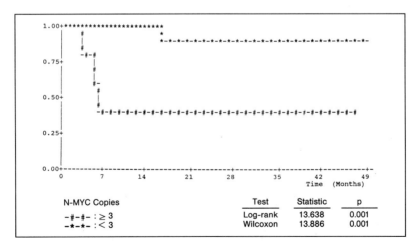

Fig. 2. Progression free survival of 25 Nb advanced stages (III & IV) by N-myc copy number in patients ≤1 year (by Kaplan-Meier method).

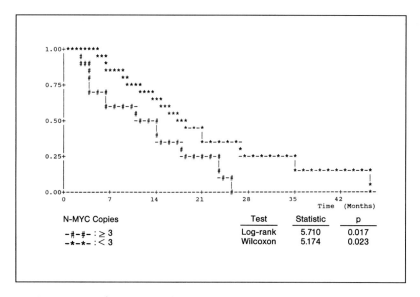

Fig. 3. Progression free survival of 32 Nb advanced stages (III & IV) by N-myc copy numbers in patients ≥1 year (by Kaplan-Meier method).

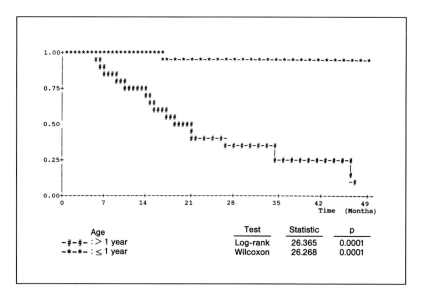

Fig. 4. Progression free survival of Nb advanced stages (III & IV) by age in patients with N-myc copy numbers <3 (by Kaplan-Meier method).

nal clinical, biochemical and molecular parameters may help to better define the prognosis and the nature of the disease(s). In particular, amplification of the N-myc oncogene was detected frequently in advanced cases of neuroblastoma in a large USA series [4] and shown to have a strong predictive value (of poor prognosis), over and above clinical staging [4].

In the present series, amplified Nb cases show a shorter PFS than non-amplified [4, 5, 15, 16]. An unexpected observation emerged when the present series (stage III, IV) was stratified by NMA (or by age at onset). While PFS of infants is strongly dependent on NMA PFS of non-amplified infant cases is significantly better than non-infants. Further data are needed to confirm and to interpret such an age effect.

Furthermore, 12 patients in this series were not included in the PFS analysis, because DNA samples at onset were not available, and 5 of these relapsing subjects showed NMA. If indeed the N-myc copy number is constant throughout the clinical course of the disease [31, 32], the fact that a high proportion of amplified cases occurs among relapsing cases (with short PFS) represents further evidence for NMA being associated with poor prognosis.

In particular the prevalence of amplified cases among infants in this series is comparable to elder children's [2], although the former age group generally displays a better prognosis [14]. Furthermore, the overall propor-

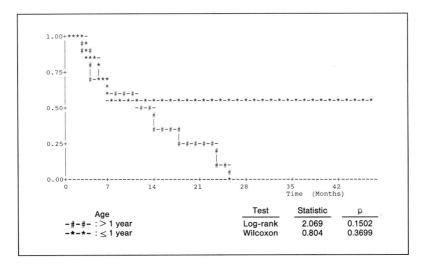

Fig. 5. Progression free survival of Nb advanced stages (III & IV) by age in patients with N-myc copy number ≥ 3 (by Kaplan-Meier method).

tion of amplified cases is lower in our series than those in the USA and Japan [4, 5]. On the other hand, long PFS in the presence of NMA has been detected in 2 out of 5 stage IV– S cases [5, 16]. The possibility of different patterns of Nb in different countries underlying the observed discrepancies cannot be ruled out [39].

The association between NMA and a less differentiated histology is worthy of further investigations, also considering the finding that N-myc expression is inversely correlated with cellular maturation in the same individual [17, 18]. Moreover, experimental data support this hypothesis: In fact, in-vitro studies showed that decreased expression of N-myc is associated with drug-induced morphological differentiation of human Nb [40, 41].

The strong correlation detected by us in a previous study on 51 Italian cases between NMA and size of the primary tumor [39] was not confirmed, and was probably attributable to a selection bias.

As for biochemical variables, excretion of VMA becomes significantly associated with N-myc only in the elder children group (age at diagnosis ≥ 1 year). The significance of this fact as a diagnostic-prognostic indicator needs further study. Previous reports [42, 43] showed catecholamine urinary excretion to be higher in patients with N-myc single copy. Such a negative correlate suggests the tumor cells of the elder children to be biochemically more immature. VMA is a late metabolite of the catecholamines' pathway, and increased levels of VMA denote cell maturation and favourable prognosis [44].

Furthermore, two enzymatic activities (NSE and LDH) appear positively correlated with NMA: NSE is considered a specific marker for neuroectodermal committed cells [19], while high LDH activity is characteristic of metabolic alterations in neoplastic cells [20, 45]. It must be noted, however, that such correlations not only are absent in infants, but they are reversed, as though the biological significance of N-myc expression may depend on the proliferation-differentiation status of the cells involved.

No correlation was found between serum ferritin levels, an important prognostic marker [46], and NMA both in the whole group and in infants.

The following conclusions are tentative, due to the small number of cases available for analysis so far. The significance of NMA as a factor of tumor progression requires further investigation, for which the study of correlations with other biological markers of malignancies may provide some clues. The different patterns of such markers found in infants and in elder children may help both to refine the predictive value of N-myc as a prognostic indicator, and to understand the natural history of the tumors that bear the name of Neuroblastoma.

Summary

In the period from January, 1984, to December, 1988, 107 neuroblastoma (Nb) fresh tumors (including 53 from patients less than 1 year old at diagnosis) were studied for N-myc amplification (NMA). In addition, NMA was correlated with other biological and clinical variables of prognostic significance. These variables included: Clinical stage [1, 2], histologic grading [3], urinary excretion of vanillylmandelic acid (VMA) and homovanillic acid (HVA), serum levels of ferritin (Fer), neuron-specific enolase (NSE) and lactic dehydrogenase (LDH), and volume (Vol) of the primary tumor. These correlations were evaluated in the whole group and by stratifying the sample by age (cut-off, 1 year).

N-myc was amplified in 7/53 Nb < 1 year (0/4 stage I, 0/8 stage II, 2/16 stage III, 3/13 stage IV, and 2/12 stage IV-S) and in 12/54 Nb $\geq$ 1 year (0/5 stage I, 0/5 stage II, 5/11 stage III, 7/32 stage IV, and 0/1 stage IV-S). The overall prevalence of NMA is significantly lower than those reported by Seeger et al. in USA [4] and by Tsuda et al. in Japan [5]. In the whole sample, NMA is related to a worse prognosis.

Analysis of the joint distribution of N-myc and histology [3] did not reveal any significant correlation between these two variables. Among tumor markers analyzed, low levels of VMA and high levels of serum NSE and LDH were significantly associated with NMA in elder children, while such correlations were lost in infants.

While the value of NMA as a prognostic indicator is confirmed by the present study, it needs some qualification. The significance of NMA as a factor of tumor progression requires further investigation, for which the study of correlations with other biological markers of malignancy may provide some clues. The different patterns of such markers found in infants and in elder children may help both to refine the predictive value of N-myc as a prognostic indicator, and to understand the natural history of Nb.

Acknowledgement

This work was supported by grant 871703 F, Ricerca Finalizzata, G. Gaslini Children's Hospital, and by Associazione Italiana per la Ricerca sul Cancro (AIRC).

References

1   Evans AE, D'Angio GJ, Randolph J: A proposed staging for children with neuroblastoma. Cancer 1971;27:374–378.
2   De Bernardi B, Rogers D, Carli M, Madon E, De Laurentis T, Bagnulo S, Di Tullio MT, Paolucci G, Pastore G: Localized neuroblastoma. Surgical and pathological staging. Cancer 1987;60:1066–1072.

3   Mäkinen J: Microscopic pattern as a guide to prognosis of neuroblastoma. Cancer 1972;29:1637–1646.

4   Seeger RC, Brodeur GM, Sather H, Dalton A, Siegel SE, Wong KY, Hammond D: Association of multiple copies of the N-myc oncogene with rapid progression of neuroblastomas. N Engl J Med 1985;313:1111–1116.

5   Tsuda T, Obara M, Hirano H, Gotoh S, Kubomura S, Higashi K, Kuroiwa A, Nagakawara A, Nagahara N, Shimizu K: Analysis of N-myc amplification in relation to disease stage and histologic types in human neuroblastomas. Cancer 1987;60:820–826.

6   Isaacs H Jr: Congenital and neonatal malignant tumors. A 28-year experience at Children's Hospital of Los Angeles. Am J Pediatr Hematol Oncol 1987;9:121–129.

7   Miller RW, Fraumeni JF Jr, Hill JA: Neuroblastoma: Epidemiologic approach to its origin. Am J Dis Child 1968;115:253–261.

8   Knudson AG Jr, Meadows AT: Developmental genetics of neuroblastoma. J Natl Cancer Inst 1976;57:675–682.

9   Sansone R, Strigini P: Genetic epidemiology of neuroblastoma and retinoblastoma and cellular oncogenes, in Tonini GP, Massimo L, Cornaglia-Ferraris P (eds): Oncogenes and pediatric tumors. London, Harwood, 1988, pp 52–95.

10   Kramer S, Ward E, Meadows AT, Malone K: Medical and drug risk factors associated with neuroblastoma: A case control study. J Natl Cancer Inst 1987;78:797–804.

11   Knudson AG Jr, Meadows AT: Regression of neuroblastoma IV–S: A genetic hypothesis. N Engl J Med 1980;302:1254–1255.

11a Brodeur GM, Fong CT: Molecular biology and genetics of human neuroblastoma. Cancer Genet Cytogenet 1989;41:153–174.

11b Martinsson T, Weith A, Cziebluch C, Schwab M: Chromosome 1 deletions in human neuroblastomas: Generation and fine mapping of microclones from the distal 1p region. Genes, Chromosomes & Cancer 1989;1:67–78.

12   Brodeur GM, Sekhon GS, Goldstein NN: Chromosomal aberrations in human neuroblastomas. Cancer 1977;40:2256–2263.

12a Fong CT, Dracopoli NC, White PS, Merril PT, Griffith RC, Housman DE, Brodeur GM: Loss of heterozigosity for the short arm of chromosome 1 in human neuroblastomas: Correlations with N-myc amplification. Proc Natl Acad Sci USA 1989; 86:3753–3757.

13   Bartram CR, Berthold F: Amplification and expression of the N-myc gene in neuroblastoma. Eur J Pediatr 1987;146:162–165.

14   Verdona G, Tonini GP: N-myc amplification in neuroblastoma and relation with classical prognostic factors of the disease, in Tonini GP, Massimo L, Cornaglia-Ferraris P (eds): Oncogenes in pediatric tumors. London, Harwood, 1988, pp 11–30.

15   Nakagawara A, Ikeda K, Tsuda T, Higashi K: N-myc oncogene amplification and prognostic factors of neuroblastoma in children. J Pediatr Surg 1987;22:895–898.

16   Nakagawara A, Ikeda K, Tsuda T, Higashi K, Okabe T: Amplification of the N-myc oncogene in stage II and IVS neuroblastoma may be a prognostic indicator. J Pediatr Surg 1987;22:415–418.

17   Nisen PD, Waber PG, Rich MA, Pierce S, Garvin JR, Gilbert F, Lanzkow P: N-myc RNA expression in neuroblastoma. J Natl Cancer Inst 1988;80:1633–1637.

18   Schwab M, Ellison J, Busch M, Roseneau W, Varmus HE, Bishop JM: Enhanced expression of the human gene N-myc consequent of amplification of DNA may con-

tribute to malignant transformation of neuroblastoma. Proc Natl Acad Sci USA 1984; 81:4940–4944.

19 Talarico D, Rosso R, Fognani C, Paulli M, Peverali AF, Solcia E, Della Valle G: Detection of N-myc oncogene mRNA in human neuroblastoma by in situ hybridization, in Tonini GP, Massimo L, Cornaglia-Ferraris P (eds): Oncogenes in pediatric tumors. London, Harwood, 1988, pp 31–51.

20 Grady-Leopardi E, Schwab M, Albin A, Roseneau W: Detection of N-myc oncogene expression in human neuroblastoma by in situ hybridization and blot analysis: Relationship to clinical outcome. Cancer Res 1987;46:3196–3199.

21 Tonini GP, Verdona G, De Bernardi B, Sansone R, Massimo L, Cornaglia-Ferraris P: N-myc amplification in a patient with stage IV–S neuroblastoma. Am J Ped Hematol Oncol 1987;9:8–10.

22 Cornaglia-Ferraris P, Tonini GP: Letter to the Editor. Am J Pediatr Hematol Oncol 1988;10:182.

22a Haas D, Ablin AR, Miller C, Zogor S, Matthay KK: Complete pathologic maturation and regression of stage IVS neuroblastoma without treatment. Cancer 1988; 62:818–825.

23 Cohn SL, Herst CV, Maurer HS, Rosen ST: N-myc amplification in an infant with stage IVS neuroblastoma. J Clin Oncol 1987;5:1441.

24 Christiansen H, Francke F, Bartram C, Adolph S, Rudolph B, Harbott J, Reiter A, Lampert F: Evolution of tumor cytogenetic aberrations and N-myc oncogene amplification in a case of disseminated neuroblastoma. Cancer Genet Cytogenet 1987;26:235:244.

25 Sansone R, Callea F, Tonini GP, Cornaglia-Ferraris P: N-myc amplification and good prognosis in two IV–S neuroblastomas. Clin Genet 1988;34:414 (Abst).

26 Maniatis T, Fritsch EF, Sambrook J: Molecular cloning. A laboratory manual. New York, Cold Spring Harbor Laboratory, 1982.

27 Verdona G, Garaventa A, De Bernardi B, Sansone R, Di Martino D, Cornaglia-Ferraris P, Tonini GP: N-myc amplification in neuroblastoma III and IV stages: Relations with other tumor markers of disease. J Tumor Mark Oncol 1986;1:105–110.

28 Scarpa S, Dominici C, Grammatico P, Del Porto G, Raschellà G, Castello M, Forni G, Modesti A: Establishment and characterization of a human neuroblastoma cell line. Int J Cancer 1989;43:645–651.

29 Pession A, Badiali M, Piratsu M, Treré D, Pianca C: Stato di avanzamento delle indagini di biologia molecolare nell' ambito dello studio integrato sul neuroblastoma. Atti del XIV Congr Nazionale A.I.E.O.P., Perugia, 8–10 Maggio 1987, pp. 199–202.

30 Rosner B: Fundamentals of biostatistics: Boston, Duxbury Press, 1982, pp 382–395.

31 Brodeur GM, Hayes A, Green AA, Casper JT, Wasson J, Wallach S, Seeger RC: Consistent N-myc copy number in simultaneous or consecutive neuroblastoma samples from sixty individual patients. Cancer Res 1987;47:4248–4253.

32 Tonini GP, Verdona G, Garaventa A, Cornaglia-Ferraris P: Antiblastic treatment does not affect N-myc gene amplification in neuroblastoma. Anticancer Res 1987; 7:729–732.

33 Brodeur GM, Seeger RC: Gene amplification in human neuroblastomas: Basic mechanisms and clinical implications. Cancer Genet, Cytogenet 1986;19:101–111.

34 Cowell JK: Double minutes and homogeneously staining regions: Gene amplification in mammalian cells. Ann Rev Genet 1982;16:21–59.

35   Roberts JM, Buck LB, Axel R: A structure for amplified DNA. Cell 1983;33:53–63.

36   Dixon WJ: BMDP statistical software. Berkeley, University of California Press, 1985; pp 557–575.

37   Mantel N: Evaluation of survival data and two new rank order statistics arising in its consideration. Cancer Chemother Rep 1966;50:163–170.

38   Breslow N: A generalized Kruskal-Wallis test for comparing k samples subjects to unequal patterns of censorship. Biometrika 1975;57:579–594.

39   Sansone R, Di Martino D, Fontana V, Marchese N, Lanino E, Strigini P, Cornaglia-Ferraris P, Tonini GP: Evaluation of N-myc copy number and its correlation with other prognostic indicators in neuroblastoma. Clin Chem Enzymol Comms 1990;2:221–226.

40   Thiele CT, Reynolds CP, Israel MA: Decreased expression of N-myc precedes retinoic acid-induced morphological differentiation of human neuroblastoma. Nature 1985;313:404–406.

41   Amatruda TT III, Sidell N, Ranyard J, Koeffler HP: Retinoic acid treatment of human neuroblastoma cells is associated with decreased N-myc expression. Biochem Biophys Res Comms 1985;126:1189–1195.

42   Nakagawara A, Ikeda K: N-myc oncogene amplification and catecholamine metabolism in children with neuroblastoma. Lancet 1987;1:559.

43   Tonini GP, Verdona G, Devoto M, Sansone R, Cornaglia-Ferraris P: N-myc oncogene amplification and catecholamine metabolism in patients with neuroblastoma. Lancet 1987;2:795.

44   Siegel SE, Laug WE: Initial urinary catecholamine metabolites and prognosis in neuroblastoma. Pediatrics 1978;62:77–87.

45   Evans AE, D'Angio GJ, Propert K, Anderson J, Hann H WL: Prognostic factors in neuroblastoma. Cancer 1987;59:1853–1859.

46   Quinn JJ, Altmann AJ, Frantz CN: Serum lactic dehydrogenase an indicator of tumor activity in neuroblastoma. J Pediat 1980;97:89–95.

Dr. Gian Paolo Tonini, Pediatric Oncology Research Laboratory,
Giannina Gaslini Children's Hospital, Largo G. Gaslini 5, I-16148 Genova (Italy)

Contrib Oncol. Basel, Karger, 1990, vol 41, pp 153–159.

Fragile Sites Expression in Neuroblastoma Patients and their Parents

A Comparison Between Patients Younger than 1 Year and Older

P. Vernole, B. Tedeschi, C. Pianca, B. Nicoletti

Department of Public Health and Cell Biology, 2nd University of Rome, Italy

Zusammenfassung

Bei 20 Kindern mit Neuroblastom (davon 9 Säuglinge) und deren Eltern wurden Chromosomenanalysen aus dem peripheren Blut durchgeführt. Die Chromosomenbrüchigkeit («breaks», «gaps», % beeinflußter Zellen) wurde durch Aphidicolinzusatz induziert. Eine höhere Chromosomenbrüchigkeit im Vergleich zu normalen altersentsprechenden Kontrollen fand sich bei Neuroblastom-Patienten (und auch bei deren Eltern). Eine geringe höhere Brüchigkeit wurde bei über 1 Jahr alten im Vergleich zu unter 1 Jahr alten Patienten gesehen. Der Unterschied war jedoch nicht statistisch signifikant.

Introduction

Chromosomal fragile sites (FS) are specific points on chromosomes that undergo breakage at an increased frequency under certain culture conditions. Fragile sites have been classified according to their frequency in the human population as rare, once also called hereditary, and common. Common fragile sites can be induced in lymphocytes from all individuals by a variety of chemicals like the antagonists of folic acid, aphidicolin, azacytidine and bromodeoxyuridine [1]. The biological significance of common fragile sites is not known.

Some FS have been localized to bands containing also recurrent breakpoints specific for some tumors and/or oncogenes [1–4]. However, the meaning of FS in cancer is still under debate [5]. Recently we have shown an increased expression of common FS induced by aphidicolin (APC), a specific inhibitor of DNA polymerase alfa, in patients affected by neuroblastoma (NB) [6].

Most neuroblastoma cases are sporadic, but in a few families there are more affected subjects. On this ground, Knudson and Strong formulated a genetical hypothesis for NB as for other paediatric tumors. In the hereditary cases a first mutation, genic or a small chromosomal deletion, might be inherited from one parent, and a successive mutation in a cell from a specific tissue would cause the development of the tumor [7]. In retinoblastoma a specific chromosomal aberration was found: The deletion 13q14 [8], while no chromosomal aberration was inherited together with the tumor in all NB patients examined [9].

We have extended our studies on FS in NB patients to the parents of 20 of them.

It is known that prognosis in neuroblastoma is linked to different parameters: One of them is the age of the patient at tumor onset [10, 11]. On this ground, we have divided the patients we studied and their parents in two groups, according to the age of the child at diagnosis, i.e. children younger than 1 year or older. Statistical analysis was used to test the possibility that the two groups may have a different sensitivity to aphidicolin.

Materials and Methods

Subjects

We examined 20 children affected by NB. 9 were younger than 1 year and the other 11 were older. In the first group, according to Evans' classification [10], one patient had stage II tumor, four stage III, three stage IV, one stage IVs. In the second group one child had stage II NB, two stage III and all the others stage IV. Personal data of the patients are shown in table 1. We also examined the parents of these children. In two cases (families 7 and 9 of the second group), only the mother was available.

Cell cultures

Whole peripheral blood was cultured in RPMI 1640, 10 % fetal calf serum and 2 % phytohemagglutinin (PHA-m, Difco) at 37°C for 72 h. 24 h before harvesting, APC (0.12 uM) was added to induce fragile sites. After an incubation of 2 h with 0.2 ug/ml colchicine, chromosome preparations and G-banding were obtained by standard methods. 50–100 metaphases from untreated and APC-treated cultures were analyzed to evaluate the number of aberrations (breaks and gaps) per cell (AB/C) and the percentage of damaged cells (cells containing at least one aberration, % DC).

We have compared data from NB patients and of their parents, with healthy subjects matched for age. Statistical analysis was performed using the normal standardized deviate, a good substitute of Student's t test when the single variances are different, and the χ^2 test on the number of damaged cells.

Results

The mean number of aberrations per cell (0.112) and of the percentage of damaged cells (0.116) in untreated cultures from NB patients were significantly higher, according to the normal standardized deviate evaluation (p < 0.01) than those found in healthy children (0.051 and 0.047). The differences were still more significant when considering APC-treated cultures. AB/C and % DC were respectively 0.677 and 0.440 in NB children and 0.190 and 0.154 in control children. To test the hypothesis that age at tumor onset may be related to sensitivity to APC, we have also considered NB children younger or older than one year separately. Both groups showed values significantly different from those of healthy children. We also compared the two groups among themselves. Data are shown in table 2. The mean value of AB/C in patients older than one year was 0.763, while in NB younger

Table 1. Personal data of the analyzed NB patients

Patients younger than one year				Patients older than one year			
Patient no.	Sex/Age*	Evans' stage	Previous therapy	Patient no.	Sex/Age*	Evans' stage	Previous therapy
1	M/0m	IV	no	1	M/15m	III	no
2	M/11m	IV	no	2	M/36m	IV	yes
3	F/0m	IVs	no	3	M/25m	III	yes
4	F/4m	III	yes	4	M/13m	IV	no
5	F/1m	II	yes	5	M/79m	IV	yes
6	F/8m	III	yes	6	F/26m	IV	no
7	M/11m	III	yes	7	F/15m	IV	no
8	F/10m	III	yes	8	F/35m	IV	no
9	F/11m	IV	yes	9	F/156m	IV	no
				10	M/108m	II	yes
				11	M/36m	IV	yes

* at diagnosis

than one year was only 0.584. However, the differences were not significant according to the normal standardized deviate.

Also, parents of NB patients showed values higher than those found in normal controls of the same age range. In untreated cultures, the mean value of AB/C were 0.073 and the % DC 0.066, while the means of controls were 0.045 and 0.042. However, the evaluation of the normal standardized deviate gave probabilities respectively of 0.04 and 0.07, values close to the limits of significativity. After APC treatment the differences became highly significant ($p < 0.01$). Parents group had a mean value of AB/C of 0.393 and a % DC of 0.306, while control values were 0.202 and 0.166.

The parents were divided in two groups according to the age of their affected child at diagnosis. Data are shown in table 2. No significant differences were found among the two groups. Then we compared each parents group with that of healthy adults.

The group of parents of children younger than 1 year showed a highly significant hypersensitivity only after APC treatment. However, when the group of parents of children older than one year was compared to the control group, chromosomal fragility was significantly higher ($p < 0.05$) even in untreated cultures.

Table 2. Mean values of aberrations per cell and of damaged cells in untreated and APC-treated cultures from NB patients younger or older than 1 year and their parents and comparison of parents groups with adult controls

	Untreated cultures		APC-treated cultures	
	AB/C	% DC	AB/C	% DC
NB patients < 1	0.129	0.120	0.584	0.419
NB patients > 1	0.116	0.115	0.763	0.467
	u=0.13	u=0.05	u=0.99	u=0.91
	p=0.89	p=0.96	p=0.32	p=0.36
Parents of NB < 1	0.061	0.053	0.360	0.277
Parents of NB > 1	0.087	0.077	0.472	0.320
	u=0.34	u=0.05	u=1.01	u=0.50
	p=0.73	p=0.96	p=0.31	p=0.61
Parents of NB < 1	u=0.85	u=0.55	u=3.52	u=3.72
versus controls	p=0.39	p=0.58	p < 0.001	p < 0.001
Parents of NB > 1	u=2.31	u=2.00	u=5.00	u=5.35
versus controls	p=0.04	p=0.05	p < 0.001	p < 0.001

u: normal standardized deviate; p: probability

Because of the heterogeneity in sensitivity to APC of NB parents, we have also considered each subject independently. Figure 1 shows the values of AB/C after APC treatment in all families. The first graph refers to families of NB patients younger than one year at diagnosis, while the second one

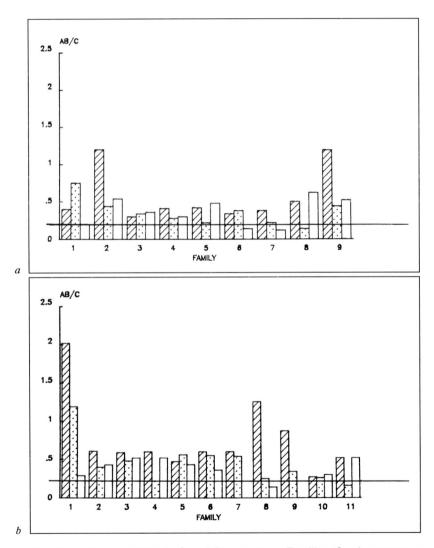

*Fig 1.*Aberrations/cell (AB/C) after APC treatment. *a.* Families of patients younger than one year. *b.* Families of patients older than one year. The horizontal line represents the AB/C mean value of control adults (0.202).

concerns the other group. The horizontal line represents the mean value of healthy adults.

Within the first group, five families have both parents showing values higher than the mean of controls. In the second group, 6 couples of parents have values higher than the mean, like the only available parent in families 7 and 9. In the remaining three families only one parent shows increased sensitivity to APC.

Discussion

Our results confirm previous data on the spontaneous chromosomal fragility of NB patients and of their hypersensitivity to APC treatment [6]. This hypersensitivity was found also in lymphocyte cultures from most NB parents. These data seem to confirm the hypothesis that the increased inducibility of FS in NB patients is a constitutional, inherited feature, not acquired after tumor development. However, for the moment we cannot say if the possible inheritance of hypersensitivity to APC may be related in any way to the transmission of a predisposition to this tumor. Because of the different clinical characteristics of neuroblastomas arisen in the first months of life or later [10, 11], we focused our attention on the possible differences in fragile sites induction among children younger or older than one year at tumor diagnosis and among their parents. A spontaneous chromosomal fragility seems to be present, not only in NB patients, but also in the parents of those of them older than one year. While parents of the other group do not differ significantly from controls, the data are still too few to determine whether there are really important differences among the two groups of parents. We will have to analyze a larger number of families.

After APC treatment, both children younger than one year and their parents showed mean values of AB/C and the % DC lower than those found in older children and their parents. However, the differences were never significant (p always >0.30). Therefore it seems that hypersensitivity to APC is a characteristic common to all neuroblastomas. Nevertheless, because of the differences we found, we cannot exclude at the moment that age at tumor diagnosis might be related to a different sensitivity to APC. We propose to extend our studies to a larger number of patients to clarify this possible relation and to analyze also other parameters, like stage of the tumor, sex, follow up and so on, that might be connected to sensitivity to APC.

Summary

Chromosome analyses from the peripheral blood were carried out in 20 children with neuroblastoma, of whom 9 were infants. Parents were included in the study. Chromosome breakage (breaks, gaps; % of damaged cells) was induced by addition of aphidicolin. A higher chromosomal fragility was found in neuroblastoma patients (and also in their parents) as compared to age-matched controls. A somewhat higher fragility was seen in patients over 1 year as compared to patients under 1 year of age. The difference was, however, not statistically significant.

References

1   Berger R, Bloomfield CD, Sutherland GR: Report of the committee on chromosome rearrangements in neoplasia and on fragile sites. Cytogenet Cell Genet 1985;40: 490–535.

2   Hecht F, Glover TW: Cancer chromosome breakpoints and common fragile sites induced by aphidicolin. Cancer Genet Cytogenet 1984;13:185–188.

3   Yunis JJ, Soreng AL: Constitutional fragile sites and cancer. Science 1984;226: 1199–1204.

4   De Brakeleer M, Smith B, Lin CC: Fragile sites and structural rearrangements in cancer. Hum Genet 1985;69:112–116.

5   Cytogenet. Cell Genet. Monographic issue 38, 1988.

6   Vernole P, Tedeschi B, Caporossi D, Nicoletti B: Common fragile sites and human cancer. A study on lymphocytes from neuroblastoma patients. Cancer Genet Cytogenet 1988;36:13–26.

7   Knudson AG, Strong LC: Mutation and cancer: Neuroblastoma and pheochromocytoma. Am J Hum Genet 1972;24:514–532.

8   Balaban G, Gilbert F, Nichols W, Meadows A, Shields J: Abnormalities of chromosome 13 in retinoblastomas from individuals with normal constitutional karyotypes. Cancer Genet Dytogenet 1982;6:213–221.

9   Moorhead PS, Evans AE: Chromosomal findings in patients with neuroblastoma, in AE Evans (ed): Advances in neuroblastoma research. New York, Raven Press 1980; pp 109–118.

10 Evans AE, D'Angio GJ, Randolph J: A proposed staging for children with neuroblastoma. Cancer 1971;27:374–378.

11 Coldman AJ, Fryer CJ, Elwood JM, Sonley MJ: Neuroblastoma: influence of age at diagnosis, stage, tumor site, and sex in prognosis. Cancer 1980;46:1896–19011.

Dr. Patrizia Vernole, Department of Public Health and Cell Biology,
Via O. Raimondo, I-00173 Roma (Italy)

Contrib Oncol. Basel, Karger, 1990, vol 41, pp 160–164.

Neuroblastoma – Family Studies as Investigated by Fragile Sites in Lymphocyte Chromosomes

B. Rudolph, F. Lampert

Oncocytogenetic Laboratory, Children's Hospital, University of Gießen, FRG

Zusammenfassung

Die Chromosomen der Blutlymphozyten von 6 Patienten mit Neuroblastom unterschiedlicher Stadien wurden unter folsäurearmen Kulturbedingungen untersucht. Bei allen Patienten konnte die Expression einer «fragile site» am Chromosom 1p13 beobachtet werden. Unter gleichen Bedingungen wurden ebenfalls die Lymphozytenchromosomen von 10 gesunden Familienmitgliedern (9 Elternteile, 1 Schwester), sowie von 9 Kontrollpersonen (4 gesund, 5 an einer Neoplasie erkrankt) analysiert. Die Familienmitglieder wurden zytogenetisch untersucht, um ihre Chromosomen auf die Expressionen der «fragile site» 1p13 zu überprüfen. 5 der 6 Mütter erwiesen sich als Überträger der «fragile site», dagegen keiner der Väter.

Fragile sites are points on chromosomes that tend to appear as nonstaining chromosome regions or chromatid gaps. A correlation between specific fragile sites and cancer breakpoints has been suggested by many authors in contradictionary reports, but no clear association was found between fragile sites and chromosomal rearrangements [8]. Fragile sites are predominantly in light G-bands (active genes), where specific chromosome rearrangements occur and where 93 % of the known oncogenes are localized [4].

In an attempt to investigate a possible relationship between fragile sites at the chromosome 1p in lymphocytes and breakpoints of chromosome 1p in neuroblastoma cancer cells, we examined the lymphocytes of children with neuroblastoma and some of their near relatives.

Methods

The heparinized peripheral blood samples of the six patients, ten family members and nine controls were cultured for 96h under folate–deprived conditions using M199 +5 % FCS (TCM 1), M199 + 5 % FCS and aphidicolin (TCM 2) or RPMI + 20 % FCS and methotrexate (TCM 3) (table 1). Aphidicolin was added in a final concentration of 0.2 μmol [3]. Methotrexate was used in a final concentration of 10^{-7}M according to a method described by Yunis [10]. The procedures of the chromosome preparation such as hypotonic treatment and fixation of the chromosomes were done by standard methods. The chromosomes were slightly treated with trypsin to reach a faint banding, and stained with Giemsa.

Table 1. Occurrence of fra1p13 in the lymphocytes of patients with neuroblastoma stage I-IV, in familymembers and controls

Individuals		1p13	breaks/anal.cells	other breaks	sex	neoplasia	TCM
88262	patient	+	2 / 10	+	f	NBL IV	3
	mother	+	4 / 50	+	f	–	3
	father	–	– / 30	+	m	–	3
86196	patient	+	11 / 70	+	f	NBL II	3
	mother	–	– / 50	+	f	–	3
87387	patient	+	2 / 43	+	m	NBL I	3
	mother	+	7 / 70	+	f	–	3
	father	–	– / 30	+	m	–	3
85479	patient	+	4 / 80	+	m	NBL III	3
	mother	+	3 / 100	+	f	–	3
TM01	patient	+	8 / 110	+	m	NBL I	1
	mother	+	6 / 80	+	f	–	3
	father	–	– / 90	+	m	–	3
ML34	mother	+	3 / 50	+	f	–	2
DL37	daughter	+	7 / 200	+	f	GN	2
DL39	daughter	+	8 / 160	+	f	–	2
Controls							
89CFRA001	healthy	–	– / 50	+	m	–	3
89CFRA002	healthy	–	– / 50	+	f	–	3
89CFRA003	healthy	–	– / 50	+	f	–	3
89CFRA004	healthy	–	– / 50	+	f	–	3
87564C001	patient	–	– / 50	+	f	ben.teratoma	3
89549C002	patient	–	– / 50	+	f	abdom.tumor	3
87NONC003	patient	–	– / 40	+	m	medullobl.	3
88NONC004	patient	+	2 / 50	+	m	melanoma	1
87NONC005	patient	–	– / 40	+	m	leukemia	3

TCM 1 M199 + 5 % FCS

   2 RPMI 1640 with methotrexate (10^{-7}mol) + 20 % FCS

   3 M199 + 5 % FCS with aphidicolin (0.2 μM)

Results

We investigated three blood samples of a so-called 'neuroblastoma family' from Salzburg (Austria) using a high resolution banding technique with methotrexate in order to detect possible aberrations at subbands of chromosome 1p. Under these conditions we induced a fragile site at chromosome 1p13.1, unknown up to that time, which we could observe in all of the three family members (M34, DL37, DL39, table 1) [7]. The index patient was a 17-years old girl with a ganglioneuroblastoma (DL37).

In further examinations, the lymphocytes of five patients with neuroblastoma (stages I–IV) and their relatives (mother and/or father) were studied under folate-deprived culture conditions (TCM 1–3) (table 1). All five patients did show the expression of a fra1p13. The parents were investigated to find out whether they had transmitted this fragile site to their children. In three of the five family studies, the fra1p13 was found in the mother's lymphocytes, but not in the father's (88262, 87387, TM01). In the other two families (86196, 85479), only the mother's lymphocytes were investigated. The expression of the fra1p13 could be observed in one case (85479). This means that, including the family from Salzburg, five out of six cytogenetically investigated mothers were carriers of the fra1p13.

One out of nine controls (88NONC004) did show a fra1p13.

Discussion

The finding of the fra1p13 is another contribution to the controversial discussion about fragile sites and chromosomal cancer breakpoints.

In our family study, we discuss the occurrence of the heritable fragile site, located at 1p13, but not the frequency of its expression. The rate of expression of the most frequent fragile sites vary among individuals as shown by Craig-Holmes [1] and in our own investigations, suggesting that a polymorphism exists at common fragile sites.

Further investigations of children with neuroblastoma revealed the presence of the fragile site 1p13 in 41 % of all cases.

An Italian group [9] confirmed the existence of the fra1p13 in children with neuroblastoma at a percentage of up to 37 %.

The high incidence of the occurrence of the aphidicolin-inducible and heritable fra1p13 does not make it easy to clarify its classification into a common or rare fragile site, and further studies will be helpful. Kaehkoenen et al. [5] studied familial transmissions of a rare fragile site. It was found in 16 to 19 (84 %) investigated families that the mother was the carrier of the fragile site, which confirms our results (83 %). On the short arm of chromosome 1, genes which may be involved in tumor development are localized, such as the oncogene Nras in 1p12 – 22 [6]. The high incidence of the breakage of chromosome 1p13 in near relatives is an indication for a familial instability in this chromosome region. Glover and Stein [2] showed in their report that fragile sites are predisposed to deletions and interchromosomal recombination measured by sister-chromatid exchanges. The demonstration of the chromosomal instability may be relevant because its location is in the same region where breakage frequently occurs in neuroblastoma cells (1p11 – 1p36).

Summary

We investigated the chromosomes of blood lymphocytes of 10 healthy family members (9 parents and 1 sister) of 6 patients with neuroblastoma of different stages as well as 9 controls (4 healthy, 5 with a neoplasia). Under folate-deficient culture conditions, all patients expressed a fragile site at chromosome 1p13. The parents were analyzed to find out whether they were carriers of the fra1p13. None of the fathers was, but 5 of the 6 examined mothers were.

Acknowledgement

This study was supported by the Deutsche Forschungsgemeinschaft (LA 185 / 7 - 2).

References

1   Craig-Holmes AP, Strong LC, Goodacre A, Pathak S: Variation in the expression of aphidicolin-induced fragile sites in human lymphocyte cultures. Hum Genet 1987; 76:134 – 137.
2   Glover TW, Stein CK: Chromosome breakage and recombination at fragile sites. Am J Hum 1988;43:265 – 273.
3   Glover TW, Berger C, Coyle J, Echo B: DNA polymerase inhibition by aphidicolin induces gaps and breaks at common fragile sites on human chromosomes. Hum Genet 1984;67:136 – 142.
4   Hecht F: Fragile sites, cancer chromosome breakpoints, and oncogenes all cluster in light G bands. Cancer Genet Cytogenet 1988;31:17 – 24.

5   Kaehkoenen M, Tengstroem C, Alitalo T, Matilainen R, Kaski M, Airaksinen E:
    Population cytogenetics of folate-sensitive fragile sites. II. Autosomal rare fragile
    sites. Hum Genet 1989;82:3–8.
6   Rabin M, Watson M, Barker PE, Ryan J, Breg WE, Rudole PH: Nras transforming
    gene maps to region p11–p13 on chromosome 1 by in situ hybridization. Cytogenet
    Cell Genet 1984;38:70–72.
7   Rudolph B, Harbott J, Lampert F: Fragile sites and neuroblastoma: Fragile site at
    1p13.1 and other points on lymphocyte chromosomes from patients and family mem-
    bers. Cancer Genet Cytogenet 1988;31:83–94.
8   Sutherland GR, Simmers RH: No statistical association between common fragile
    sites and nonrandom chromosome breakpoints in cancer cells. Cancer Genet Cyto-
    genet 1988;31:9–15.
9   Vernole P, Tedeschi B, Caporossi D, Nicoletti B: Fragile site 1p13.1 in neuroblastoma
    patients. Cancer Genet Cytogenet 1989;40:135–136.
10 Yunis JJ: New chromosome techniques in the study on human neoplasia. Hum
    Pathol 1981;12:540–549.

Prof. Dr. Fritz Lampert, Universitäts-Kinderpoliklinik,
Feulgenstraße 12, D-6300 Gießen (FRG)

Contrib Oncol. Basel, Karger, 1990, vol 41, pp 165–173.

Soft Tissue Sarcomas in Infants Less than 1 Year Old: Experience of the Italian Cooperative Study RMS-79[1]

M. Carli, P. Grotto, G. Perilongo, L. Cordero di Montezemolo,
G. Cecchetto, B. De Bernardi, G. Deb, M.T. Di Tullio, S. Bagnulo,
M. LoCurto, A. Mancini, L. Andrello, G. Sotti, G. Masarotto

Department of Pediatrics, University of Padua, Italy

Zusammenfassung

18 Säuglinge wurde in der Italienischen Kooperativstudie RMS-79 registriert und behandelt. 10 Patienten hatten ein Rhabdomyosarkom (7 ein «embryonales», 3 ein «alveoläres», 8 andere Weichteilsarkome (Fibrosarkom, Haemangiosarkom und andere). Die Kopf-Halsregion war in 5 Fällen, die Extremitäten in 2, die Orbita in 1, der Urogenitaltrakt in 1 und andere Stellen in 9 Fällen der Ausgangsort. Die Behandlung durch Operation (Bestrahlung) und Chemotherapie (Cyclophosphamid, Vincristin, Adriamycin, Actinomycin D) resultierte in einer 5-Jahres- ereignisfreien bzw. Gesamt-Überlebensrate von 53 % bzw. 67 % (im Vergleich zu 45 % bzw. 49 % bei älteren Patienten).

Soft tissue sarcomas (STS) are the fifth most common cancer in children under 15 years of age, following acute leukemia, central nervous system tumors, lymphoma and neuroblastoma [1].

However, in children younger than 1 year of age, STS rank fourth following neuroblastoma, leukemia and kidney tumors, with annual incidence of 17.8 cases per million live births [2].

The relative proportion of STS in infants has been reported to vary from 11 % to 13 % of all STS observed in children less than 15 years of age [3, 4].

The clinical management of STS in infants may represent a problem due to the immaturity of important organs such as brain, lung, liver, kidney and bone and the vulnerability to the late effects of treatment.

[1] Supported by CNR Special Project 'Oncology' Contract n. 88.00569.44

Thus, some crucial questions have to be answered, and they concern mainly the type of treatment and its aggressiveness weighed against the prognosis and the possibility of significant late effects.

The aim of this report is to review the clinical characteristics and outcome of infants enrolled in the Italian cooperative study on STS (ICS – RMS 79).

Materials and Methods

Between October 1, 1979 and December 31, 1986, 18 children less than 1 year of age were enrolled in the ICS RMS-79 (three of them entered at the time of first local relapse, after a previous surgical resection). They account for 7.7 % of 234 children aged less than 15 years treated in this protocol.

Sex and age

Thirteen were male and 5 female. The median age at diagnosis was 4 months. Five tumors (27 %) were probably of congenital origin, since detected in the first month of life; six infants were aged between 1 to 6 months and 7 between 7 to 12 months at the time of diagnosis (table 1).

Histology

All histological material of the 18 cases of this report were reviewed by the ICS Pathology Committee (as it was for 176 out of 234 cases registered in the study).

Table 1. Age distribution of patient younger than 1 year in ICS RMS-79

Age in months	No. of patients
1	5
2	1
3	3
4	–
5	1
6	1
7	1
8	1
9	2
10	1
11	2

Rhabdomyosarcoma accounted for 10 cases (55,5 %), (embrional 7, and alveolar 3) and other STS (NRSTS) for 8 (45.5 %), including 4 fibrosarcoma, 2 haemangiosarcoma, 1 malignant schwannoma and 1 ectomesenchymoma (table 2). In the older group of children the frequency of RMS and NRSTS was 77 % and 23 % respectively.

Primary site and stage

Primary sites were head/neck in 5 cases, orbit in 1, genito-urinary tract in 1, extremity in 2 and other sites in 9 (table 3).

According to the IRS grouping system [5], 5 were in clinical group I, 4 in group II, 8 in group III and 1 in group IV (table 4).

Treatment

Patients had primary surgery whenever a conservative surgical excision was possible. All others received a three month primary chemotherapy (pCT) with Vincristine, Actino-mycin D and Cyclophosphamide (VAC) [6], aimed to reduce the tumor mass and to test its efficacy in STS. Surgery was subsequently employed to eradicate residual tumor.

Radiotherapy (RT) was scheduled for macro/microscopical residual disease. Maintenance CT consisted of alternate courses of CAV (Cyclo, VCR and Adriamycin) and VAC. The whole treatment lasted 12 months or 18 months for patients in groups III-IV, or with alveolar RMS or extremity primary [7].

Table 2. Pathologic subgroups in infants younger than 1 year of age and in older children in ICS RMS-79

Pathologic type	< 1 year (n=18) (%)	1–15 years (n=158 %) (%)
Rhabdomyosarcoma	10 (55.5)	123 (77)
embrional	7 (70)	94 (76)
alveolar	3 (30)	29 (23)
Non RMS STS	8 (45.5)	35 (23)
fibrosarcoma	4	5
haemangiosarcoma	2	1
ectomesenchimoma	1	–
M. Schwannoma	1	4
PNET	–	6
SARCOMA NOS	–	3
synovial S.	–	3
E.O. Ewing	–	5
others	–	8

Drug dosage was calculated according to body weight, which represents a 30–50 % reduction of dosage based on body surface area (BSA). A further reduction to 1/3 of the theoretical BSA dose was utilized in very small infants.

Results

Treatment schedule was not uniform: It included surgery (S) alone (1 patient), CT alone (4), S+CT (9), S+CT+RT (1) and CT+RT (3); thus, 17 infants received CT. Eight patients with an unresectable tumor at diagnosis received CT as first therapy: Three complete responses (CR) were achieved in 3 infants with RMS and 3 partial response (PR) in 2 with RMS and 1 with haemangiosarcoma (CR+PR=77 %). The other 2 (1 RMS and 1 fibrosarcoma) failed to respond. RT was administered in 5 infants with residual

Table 3. Primary site of STS in infants younger than 1 year of age and in older patients in ICS RMS-79

Primary site	< 1 year (%)	1–15 years (%)
Orbit	1 (5.5)	24 (11)
Head / neck	5	53
nonPM	3 (17)	19 (9)
PM	2 (11)	34 (16)
Extremity	2 (11)	33 (15)
Genito-urinary	1 (5.5)	38 (18)
Other sites	9 (50)	68 (31)
Total	18	216

Table 4. Clinical groups in infants younger than 1 year of age and in older children in ICS RMS-79

Clinical group	< 1 year (%)	1–15 years (%)
I	5 (28)	42 (19)
II	4 (22)	33 (15)
III	8 (44)	112 (52)
IV	1 (5)	29 (13)
Total	18	216

disease after surgery or initial pCT (1 received RT for an uncompleted surgical excision of a local relapse): CR was obtained in 3 patients receiving more than 40 Gy.

In conclusion, sixteen infants (88.8 %) achieved CR status either with CT+S+RT (15 cases) or surgery alone (1 case). Two patients achieved a PR and an objective response as best response.

The actuarial 5-year event-free and overall survival rates estimated by Kaplan-Meier method, are 53 % and 67 % respectively (compared to 45 % and 49 % respectively in older children (fig. 1, 2).

Currently, 12 infants are alive without evidence of disease with a follow-up ranging from 31 to 118 months (median 51 mos); according to the histological subtype, 8 out 10 patients with RMS and 4 out 8 with NRSTS are alive; according to the clinical group, 5/5 in group I, 2/4 in group II, 5/8 in group III and 0/1 in group IV (table 5) are alive.

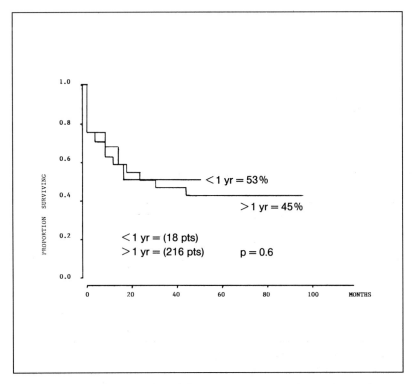

Fig. 1 Event free survival in infants less than 1 year of age and older children with STS (ICS RMS-79).

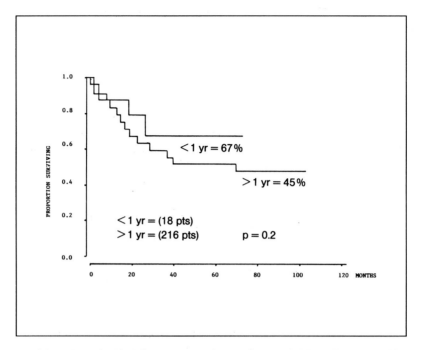

Fig. 2 Overall survival in infants less than 1 year of age and older children with STS (ICS RMS-79).

Table 5. Outcome of infants younger than 1 year of age in ICS RMS-79

Group	No.	Alive/NED	Failures (first event)				
			PD	L	L+M	M	death
I	5	5	–	–	–		–
II	4	2			1		2*
III	8	5	2	2[+]			3
IV	1	–		1			1
Total	18	12	2	3	1		6

* 1 death due to complication (pneumonia)
[+] 1 pt. alive in 2nd CR
PD = progressive disease; L = local failure; L+M = local failure + metastases;
NED = No evidence of disease

Failure

The two patients who did not achieve CR (1 RMS and 1 fibrosarcoma) died of local progressive disease.

Three local failures occurred in 2 group III patients with RMS and in 1 group IV with haemangiosarcoma; 1 infant with group II malignant schwannoma presented local recurrence plus lung metastases.

An infant, in general poor condition at presentation, died of pneumonia after the second course of CT.

Discussion

This series of 18 infants represents 7.7 % of whole STS enrolled in the ICS RMS 79 in the 7-year period of study. This frequency is similar to the one reported by Koscielniak [3] and Ragab [8] and slightly lower to the one published by Salloum [9].

In this series, NRSTS represented 45 % of all cases, a higher proportion than that observed in older children. Fibrosarcoma was the most frequent tumor of this group.

As far as clinicopathological characteristics are concerned, no major differences were observed between infants and older children. However, a higher percentage of males (72 %) was noted in infants than in the older age group (53 %).

The treatment plan adopted for these infants was the same as for older children. However, drug dosage calculation was based on body weight, which represents a 30–50 % reduction of the dosage based on BSA. Even less chemotherapy was delivered to very young infants (less than 3 months). In fact, they usually received 30 % of the theoretical dosage calculated according to BSA.

Using this drug dosage calculation, we observed few severe toxic effects; the only therapy-related death we registered occurred in a 1-month old baby in very poor general conditions at presentation, who was treated with 1/3 of the theoretical dose of chemotherapy. Other reports demonstrated the unacceptable toxicity of delivering full dose chemotherapy in infants [8, 11] and the feasibility of treating them 30 to 50 % drug dosage reduction. Adopting this 'policy', few fatal or life-threatening complications were observed in infants [3, 8–10]. This may be related to the fact that the metabolism of chemotherapeutic drugs is altered in infants younger than 1 year, particularly in the neonate [11].

The tumor response rate to pCT and the survival curves we obtained indicate that this drug dosage reduction did not affect the outcome of these infants. In fact, in our study no differences were observed, either in the response rate to pCT [6] or event free and overall survival, between infants and older children.

The lack of tumor control was the major cause of tumor failure. Apparently, in our series local tumor relapse was slightly more frequent among infants with micro- and macroscopical residual disease who did not receive RT, in comparison with those who were irradiated (3 out of 6 vs. 1 out of 4, respectively). However, other authors did not observe an increased rate of local recurrence in infants younger than 1 year of age with RMS in comparison to older children who received RT [3].

In spite of these data, it seems reasonable to recommend to limit the use of RT in infants with STS in the light of late effects of this therapeutic modality. Thus, the use of conservative radical surgery associated with chemotherapy must be encouraged. Interestingly, none of the children of our series who had radical tumor excision at presentation or after primary CT did suffer of local tumor recurrence.

In conclusion:

– Children less than 1 year old with a STS seem to have a survival rate similar to that of older children.

– Adequate CT dosage modification can avoid life-threatening complications without jeopardizing the survival rate of these infants.

– Multimodality therapy is also the treatment of choice for infants.

– The use of RT in children younger than 1 year of age must be weighed against the possibility of significant late effects, considering that a good local control of disease can be obtained with S and CT.

Summary

18 infants less than 1 year of age were enrolled in the Italian Cooperative Study RMS-79. 10 patients had Rhabdomyosarcoma (7 Embryonal, 3 Alveolar), 8 other soft tissue sarcomas (Fibrosarcoma, haemangiosarcoma and others). Head-neck was involved in 5 cases, extremities in 2, orbit in 1, genito-urinary tract in 1 and other sites in 9. Treatment by surgery, radiotherapy and chemotherapy (Cyclophosphamide, Vincristin, Adriamycin, Actinomycin D) resulted in a 5-year event-free and overall survival rate of 53 %, respectively 67 % (as compared to 45 %, resp. 49 % in older children).

References

1 Young JL Jr, Ries LG, Silverberg E, et al: Cancer incidence, survival and mortality for children younger than age 15 years. Cancer 1986;58:598–602.
2 Bader JL, Miller RW: Cancer incidence and mortality in the first year of life. Am J Dis Child 1979;133:157–159.
3 Koscielniak E, Harms D, Schmidt D, Keim M, Riehm H, Treuner J: Soft tissue sarcomas in infants younger than 1 year of age: a report of the German Soft Tissue Sarcoma Study Group (CWS-81). Med Ped Oncol 1989;17:105–110.
4 Neira C, Ninane J, Verbruggen B, Vernylen C, Cornu G: Malignancies in children less than one year old. Relative incidence and survival. SIOP XXI Meeting. Abstracts. Med Ped Oncol 1989;176:323.
5 Maurer HM: The Intergroup Rhabdomyosarcoma Study: Update Nov. 1978. Natl Cancer Inst Monogr 1981;56:61–68.
6 Carli M, Pastore G, Perilongo G, Grotto P, De Bernardi B, Ceci A, Di Tullio M, Madon E, Pianca C, Paolucci G: Tumor response and toxicity after single high-dose versus standard five-day divided-dose dactinomycin in childhood rhabdomyosarcoma. J Clin Oncol 1988;6:654–658.
7 Carli M, Guglielmi M, Grotto P, Sotti G, Perilongo G, De Bernardi B, Mancini A, Colella R, De Laurentis C, Cordero di Montezemolo L, Indolfi P, Pastore G, Masarotto G, for the STS-ICG: Rhabdomyosarcoma in childhood: A report from the italian Cooperative Study, in De Bernardi B, Kornhuber B, Massimo L, Lampert F (eds): Proceedings of the workshop on Pediatric Oncology, Genova, Nov. 13–14, 1987, p 132–138.
8 Ragab AH, Heyn R, Tefft M, Hays DN, Newton WA, Beltangady M: Infants younger than 1 year of age with rhabdomyosarcoma. Cancer 1986;58:2606–2610.
9 Salloum E, Flamant F, Rey A, Cailland JM, Friedman S, Valteau D, Lemerle J: Rhabdomyosarcoma in infants under one year of age: experience of the Institut Gustave-Roussy. Med Ped Oncol 1989;17:424–428.
10 Morgan E, Baum E, Bleslow N, Takashima J, D'Angio G: Chemotherapy related toxicity in infants treated according to the Second National Wilms' Tumor Study. J Clin Oncol 1988;6:51–55.
11 Siegel SE, Moran RG: Problems in the chemotherapy of cancer in the neonate. Am J Pediat Hematol Oncol 1981;3:287–296.
12 Cecchetto G, Pastore G, Guglielmi M, Grotto P, Boglino G, Rizzo A, Previtera C, Carli M: La chirurgia dei sarcomi delle parti molli nel primo anno di vita. X Congresso Societa' Italiana Chirurgia Oncologica (SICO). Palermo 24–27 settembre 1986. Monduzzi, p 545–548.

M. Carli, M.D., Department of Pediatrics Hematology-Oncology Division, University of Padova, Via Giustiniani 3, I-35128 Padova (Italy)